PRAISE FOR
BEING BEHELD

"In *Being Beheld*, Jordan Mason sheds new light on discussions about process and method in the field of clinical ethics. She takes us deep into the phenomenology of clinical ethics consultation and uses liturgy and ritual to analyze what kind of action ethics consultation is. She shows that theology and virtue ethics must have a substantial role in the ongoing development of clinical ethics as a profession. Mason's thinking and practical approach to a theological clinical ethics is a refreshing addition to the conversation of what the practice clinical ethics is and what it should be."

BECKET GREMMELS, System Vice President for Theology and Ethics, CommonSpirit Health

"*Being Beheld* is a deeply thoughtful and indeed revolutionary exploration of ethics consultation practices. Moving beyond the sterile application of standardized methods, this book presents a compelling argument that the search for a patient's good should be a sacred, participatory practice, open to mystery. By drawing parallels to the eucharistic liturgy, it offers a powerful new framework built on narrative, humility, and encounter. With its blend of practical case studies and clear-eyed theory, this book is essential reading for theologians, ethicists, and especially practicing health care ethics consultants."

ERICA K. SALTER, PHD, HEC-C, Associate Professor of Health Care Ethics and Pediatrics, Saint Louis University

"With clarity and urgency, Jordan Mason interrogates not only what ethics is—or is not—in contemporary applied settings like clinical ethics consultations, but also the conditions and contexts shaping those who practice it. This is essential reading for anyone seeking to understand the labor of medical ethics and clinical professionals and the worlds they are forming through that work."

ASHLEY JOHN MOYSE, Associate Professor of Bioethics, Baylor University

Being Beheld

Being Beheld

On the Liturgical Consummation of Clinical Ethics Consultation

Jordan Mason

BLOOMSBURY ACADEMIC
NEW YORK • LONDON • OXFORD • NEW DELHI • SYDNEY

BLOOMSBURY ACADEMIC

Bloomsbury Publishing Inc, 1359 Broadway, New York, NY 10018, USA
Bloomsbury Publishing Plc, 50 Bedford Square, London, WC1B 3DP, UK
Bloomsbury Publishing Ireland, 29 Earlsfort Terrace, Dublin 2, D02 AY28, Ireland

BLOOMSBURY, BLOOMSBURY ACADEMIC and the Diana logo are trademarks of
Bloomsbury Publishing Plc

First published in the United States of America 2026

Copyright © Jordan Mason, 2026

For legal purposes the Acknowledgments on p. xi constitute an extension of this copyright page.

Cover design: Diana Nuhn
Cover background artwork © iStock.om/ scotto72, hands © iStock.om/Shemelina

Excerpt from "Color Blindness, History, and the Law" by Kimberlé Williams Crenshaw, copyright © 1997; from *The House That Race Built: Black Americans, U.S. Terrain* edited by Wahneema Lubiano. Used by permission of Pantheon Books, an imprint of the Knopf Doubleday Publishing Group, a division of Penguin Random House LLC. All rights reserved.

Excerpt from *You Are What You Love* by James K. A. Smith, copyright © 2016. Used by permission of Brazos Press, a division of Baker Publishing Group. Smith, *You Are What You Love: The Spiritual Power of Habit.*, 45. All rights reserved.

Excerpt from *Under the Gaze of the Bible* by Jean-Louis Chretien, copyright © 2014. Used with permission of Fordham University Press. Permission conveyed through Copyright Clearance Center, Inc. Jean-Louis Chretien, *Under the Gaze of the Bible*, ed. John D. Caputo, trans. John Marson Dunaway, Perspectives in Continental Philosophy (New York: Fordham University Press, 2015), 41 and 42. All rights reserved.

Excerpt from *Aspects of Truth: A New Religious Metaphysics* by Catherine Pickstock, copyright © 2020. Reproduced with permission of The Licensor through PLSclear. *Aspects of Truth: A New Religious Metaphysics* (Cambridge: Cambridge University Press, 2020). All rights reserved.

Excerpt from *Addressing Patient-Centered Ethical Issues in Health Care: A Case-Based Study Guide*. Chicago, IL: ASBH. Copyright © 2017, American Society for Bioethics and Humanities. Reprinted with permission. All rights reserved.

Excerpt from "Health is Membership" from *The Art of the Commonplace: The Agrarian Essays*, copyright © 1994, 2002 by Wendell Berry. Reprinted with the permission of The Permissions Company, LLC on behalf of Counterpoint Press, counterpointpress.com. All rights reserved.

All rights reserved. No part of this publication may be: i) reproduced or transmitted in any form, electronic or mechanical, including photocopying, recording or by means of any information storage or retrieval system without prior permission in writing from the publishers; or ii) used or reproduced in any way for the training, development or operation of artificial intelligence (AI) technologies, including generative AI technologies. The rights holders expressly reserve this publication from the text and data mining exception as per Article 4(3) of the Digital Single Market Directive (EU) 2019/790.

Bloomsbury Publishing Inc does not have any control over, or responsibility for, any third-party websites referred to or in this book. All internet addresses given in this book were correct at the time of going to press. The author and publisher regret any inconvenience caused if addresses have changed or sites have ceased to exist, but can accept no responsibility for any such changes.

Library of Congress Cataloging-in-Publication Data

ISBN: HB: 979-8-2162-7867-2
PB: 979-8-2162-7866-5
ePDF: 979-8-2162-7869-6
eBook: 979-8-2162-7868-9

Typeset by Deanta Global Publishing Services, Chennai, India
Printed and bound in the United States of America

For product safety related questions contact productsafety@bloomsbury.com.

To find out more about our authors and books visit www.bloomsbury.com and sign up for our newsletters.

To Taylor Mason,
whose love daily strengthens me
for my work in the world

Contents

Acknowledgments	xi
Prelude	xiii
The Problem: Standardization of Clinical Ethics Techniques	xviii

Part I Standardized Clinical Ethics Consultation Techniques

1   What Is a Technique?   3
    Heidegger on *Techne*   3
    Heidegger's *Techne* within the Philosophy of Technology   7
    Techno-Ontology: Challenging-Forth in Clinical Ethics Consultation   13

2   What Does a Technique Do?   27
    Non-Identical Repetition   28
    Challenging-Forth and Identical Repetition   31
    Encounter and Being   36
    Ersatz Liturgies   39

3   The Four Boxes Method, Clinical Pragmatism, Bioethics Mediation, and the VA's CASES Method   47
    The Four Boxes Method   48
    Clinical Pragmatism   55
    Bioethics Mediation   62
    A Note on ASBH's Ethics Facilitation Standards   73
    The VA's CASES Method   75

4   Richard Zaner's Phenomenological Method   93
    Zaner's Phenomenological Method   94
    Foucault's Critique of Phenomenology and Other Kantian Philosophies   102
    Phenomenology's Revealing and Concealing   107

Interlude	113
CEC and the Virtue of *Phronesis*	121
Locally Building and Evaluating Techniques	124

Part II Practical Ethics as Liturgical Activity

5 The Liturgy's Participatory Ontology	135
Liturgical Ontological Revealing	139
What Participatory Ontology Does Not Mean: Rejecting Pantheism	150
Practical Ethics with a Participatory Ontology	151
6 Practices of Participation, Not Power: Clinical Ethics Consultation Techniques in a Liturgical Stance	159
Some Features of a Liturgical Stance	161
Summary	168
Postlude	171
Bibliography	181
Index	193
About the Author	195

Acknowledgments

It is humbling to think of all those who have had a hand in the development of this book. So many teachers, colleagues, and friends have helped to nurture these ideas as they have taken form in me over the years. I especially want to acknowledge those who have given me detailed feedback as the manuscript developed from its earliest stages, including my dissertation director Jeffrey P. Bishop and my dissertation committee members Kimbell Kornu, Erica K. Salter, and Catherine Pickstock. How generous you four have been toward me—intellectually generous, generous with your time, generous with your resources.

I have a number of mentors in ethics to thank for their guidance and inspiration through the years, including Andy Watts at Belmont University, David P. Gushee at Mercer University (who was also instrumental in getting this book published), and Jeffrey P. Bishop (whose influence is, of course, clearly displayed throughout); I was additionally mentored in clinical ethics by the excellent Becket Gremmels and Jay Malone. You are each exemplars. What you have taught me goes beyond knowledge—it has entered into my bones and finds its way into all my embodied and written work. Thank you.

This book would not have been possible without a wider community of scholars and practitioners who have supported not only this project but my development as an ethicist. That community includes my graduate professors at St. Louis University: Harold Braswell, Jason Eberl, Kimbell Kornu, Erica K. Salter, and Jeffrey P. Bishop. I must also acknowledge the numerous friends I made at SLU who allowed (and continue to allow) me to kick around my ideas with them and who continue to offer me support in my clinical ethics work: Amanda Berg, Andrea Thornton, Paul Riffon, Sarah Sawicki, Kirsten Dempsey, Addison Tenorio Lane, Annie Friedrich, and Jaime Konerman-Sease, among many others (the circle is wider than I deserve). The circle, of course, extends beyond SLU to friends across the country who keep me intellectual company (I think especially of Ashley John Moyse, whose writing and clear thinking fortified mine as I developed this book). I also continue to be greatly supported and edified by my ethics colleagues at Providence and in the broader world of Catholic healthcare ethics. Together, this wide community of faithful thinkers and doers keeps me tethered to both theory and practice, should I ever stray too far in either direction.

I must also heartily acknowledge the contributions of my husband, Taylor Mason, who is one of the very few people to have read every word of this manuscript in its early iterations. His feedback at every stage of the process—as well as his very material support—has seen this work to the finish line. He makes it possible for me to devote so much heart and soul (and time) to my vocation, and his engagement as an interlocutor improves all of my writing and thinking.

Finally, I would be remiss not to acknowledge the clinicians alongside whom I engage in the moral work of clinical ethics at Providence. I learn so much from observing their practice of medicine, how they discern and clarify, and how they care. And of course, the patients who continue to teach me how to be an ethicist. As my teacher Jeffrey P. Bishop wrote in the acknowledgments of his first book, "We are always students, all of us, every time we walk into a patient's room." I am honored to be their perpetual student.

Prelude

Clinical Ethics and Standardization

It is fairly obvious that treating different things the same can generate as much inequality as treating the same things differently. —Kimberlé Crenshaw[1]

In 2018, clinical ethicists Stuart G. Finder and Mark J. Bliton published a book containing a case consultation narrative titled "The Zadeh Scenario."[2] The case narrative, a real and deidentified scenario, chronicles the ethicist's (Finder's) interactions with the Zadeh/Hamadani family and their medical team. Mrs. Hamadani, the patient, is an 83-year-old woman with lung cancer whose devoted children are refusing to follow the team's recommendations to stop aggressive treatment. The case is a complicated one—involving cultural differences, a complex medical picture, many family members and physicians, and multiple ethicists—yet surprisingly, the Zadeh Scenario is not the most interesting part of Finder and Bliton's book. It is not the most interesting part of the book because, along with the case narrative, the book contains multiple peer commentaries written by other clinical ethicists on Finder's consultation process, as well as peer commentaries on those commentaries, and even another layer of peer commentaries after that. These commentaries reveal a set of assumptions carried along by the stream of contemporary clinical ethics which are rarely verbalized or interrogated, yet which determine in large part the direction the practice is heading. Finder and Bliton's book turns out to be most interesting not for what it says about the Zadeh Scenario, then, but for what it displays about clinical ethicists themselves.

By the final layer of peer commentaries, toward the end of the book, commenters begin to notice a pattern of concerns being raised in response to Finder's case narrative. Courtenay R. Bruce and Jeffrey P. Bishop independently point out that all of the responses devote at least some (and in some cases, a lot) of attention to *process* or *procedural failures* by the ethicists responding to the Zadeh Scenario. More specifically, rather than raising ethical questions about Finder's handling of the case (related to goods, values, moral outcomes, virtues, etc.), Finder's peers critique him for not conforming to the American Society for Bioethics and Humanities' (ASBH's) process recommendations. While opinions on the specifics of Finder's successes or failures in this case differ, they all have in common an insistence that his success or failure hinges on one thing: procedure. Did Finder follow ASBH's process recommendations? Did he display in his approach the ASBH's core competencies? Did he follow a method that meets ASBH approval?

Since the inception of our field, clinical ethicists have tended to have different views on the nature and purpose of clinical ethics consultation (CEC), the moral expertise and authority we can claim in the public sphere, and the types of methods appropriate for CEC.[3] These issues have garnered robust attention in the bioethics literature for decades.[4] Since the founding of the ASBH in 1998, though, divergent visions have been slowly coalescing around one vision, inscribed in, for instance, the "Core Competencies for Healthcare Ethics Consultation" (published in 1998 and 2010), a "Code of Ethics and Professional Responsibilities for Healthcare Ethics Consultants" (published in 2014), and a certification program for ethics consultants (HEC-C, launched in 2018).[5] Or if not coalescing around a single practice, since some debate remains, it may be more accurate to say divergent visions have been placed to one side as our professional body moves forward with the majority vision. While the intraprofessional debates around the nature of clinical ethics consultation, its philosophical foundations, its canon of authoritative guidance or "consensus," its moral authority, its rightful place within institutions, etc. have not been settled, ASBH's unifying work has allowed clinical ethics to continue to professionalize. Some bioethicists continue to critique the professionalization of clinical ethics; I would contend it is not professionalization itself that poses dangers to the integrity of clinical ethics. Rather, it is the standardization of our practice, particularly of our methods or techniques, that poses such a danger.

But a unified procedure is thought to be a necessary part of professionalization. One hope is that if we all follow the same standard process, the legitimacy of our (relatively new) profession can be demonstrated and communicated to our institutional settings in ways they will understand and value: repeatability, quality improvement, proper oversight, data, and metrics.[6] If processes are standardized across the profession, we think, we can show reliability and quality. We can study the efficacy of ethics in our organizations, in the same way that medical interventions are tested and studied in the controlled environment of evidence-based medicine. For example, Sharon Feldman et al. argue that

> Benchmarks against which healthcare ethics consultation (HCEC) services can assess their performance are needed. . . . This will be possible only with widespread reporting of standardized data points. . . . Given that volume-based metrics are the native language of the clinical environment, efforts to improve such metrics in the [HCEC] field through transparency and standardization are warranted.[7]

If we have an agreed-upon method or set of methods in addition to our competencies and other professional standards, then we can collect data and evidence showing the value of clinical ethics to patients, providers, and institutions.[8] In short, we can secure our presence in medical spaces, our legitimacy as professionals, and our livelihoods.

But while I suspect these institutional and professional interests play a large role in the narrowing of approaches,[9] another (perhaps more important, yet underacknowledged) reason for standardization in clinical ethics is our firm belief that there is a *right* way to do it—and we should all be meeting that benchmark. If there is a right way to do it, a normative "how" of CEC, then quality will coincide with uniformity. Because of this belief, clinical ethics has become increasingly about homogenizing right action, assuming that right action will reliably lead us to good ethical outcomes.

Right action in CEC means right methods, right techniques, for approaching medical-moral dilemmas. There is a sense that educational backgrounds, core disciplines, religious beliefs, etc., may still vary between ethicists, as long as the Core Competencies are met; the Core Competencies are aimed at the ability to carry out a certain right action of CEC. In fact, this right action of CEC is thought to ensure that *even while* educational backgrounds, core disciplines, religious beliefs, etc., *do* differ between ethicists, the result will remain the same and of high quality. In a way, uniformity of procedure is a reaction to the perceived threat of ideological diversity within our ranks.

The assumption that standardized techniques of CEC, in particular, will yield quality results has been reified in clinical ethics literature for decades, with scholars taking for granted that, "Regardless of the process [either by individual, subcommittee, or committee], an ethics consultation should *use a method* to ensure that all relevant information is gathered and analyzed before recommendations are made."[10] Emphasis on right action is operative behind mainstream opinions like

> there is a need for substantive standards for—and a clear notion of process to direct—clinical ethics consultation. It should not be the case that a service this common proceeds with no precise idea of . . . how consultations should be conducted, documented and reviewed for quality.[11]

And,

> [The] need to address this lack of an assessment tool to evaluate the approach, quality and content of [CEC], assess its long-term effects on patient care and safety, and standardise and benchmark practice is further underlined by evidence of *variations in CEC practice and [CEC] methods that will ultimately undermine the efficacy and standing of CECs as a whole.* Better understanding of how CECs meet this key role will also improve . . . quality standards and guidelines of CECs.[12]

And, "despite [ASBH] having made strides toward consensus on how ethics consultation ought to be performed, many inconsistencies exist, limiting the ability to ensure the quality of ethics consultation."[13] In short, increasing standardization of technique is the horizon of CEC because standardization is assumed to secure quality. When we encounter a case of conflict or confusion, clinical ethicists are increasingly expected to deploy a standardized, repeatable, and rationally defensible technique for working toward a recommendation and/or consensus. Whatever their differences, the peer reviewers (excluding Bishop) of Finder's Zadeh Scenario agree on this much at least. A handful of popular CEC methods exist; each has slightly different working conceptions of ethics expertise, moral justification, and ideal outcome, but all operate under the assumption that the efficacious, repeatable technique, when performed correctly, will yield the proper result.

It is this drive behind technique standardization—the assumption that uniform methods deliver high quality—that I am examining and challenging in this book. I have chosen to challenge this assumption rather than the drive for professionalization or institutional value because I believe standardization of technique *in particular* has far-reaching metaphysical and moral implications. The problem runs quite deep, I will claim—to the heart of ethical inquiry, and to the ontological heart of being itself. In the pages that follow, I will contextualize the movement toward standardized action in clinical ethics before outlining my critiques and suggestions for a better way to conceive of CEC.

But let me first zoom out. This book sits at the intersection of quite a few areas of concern. It can be succinctly described as a theology of technique for clinical ethics qua practical ethics. By practical ethics, I mean something like what Dennis Thompson describes[14]—not applied ethics (wherein external ethical theories and principles are "applied" unidirectionally to concrete problems in various domains) but rather an approach by which we allow the concrete realities of these practical contexts to revise our ethical principles and vice versa, in a circular process of continued adjustment and correction. Precisely because practical ethics has a circular movement between theory and practice, which should not be separated, this book is intended for both scholars of bioethics and practitioners of clinical bioethics. It will provide each with a theoretical grounding upon which to build a reflective practice of engagement with moral questions in healthcare, and will offer practical suggestions for such building, including several case studies in the Interlude and Part II. The book will not suggest we cease on our path of professionalizing, but rather that we attend more carefully to the integrity of our practices and avoid the pitfalls of standardizing the wrong things.

In addition to its synthesis of theory and practice, this book engages both philosophy and theology. I expect it to be taken up by those working at the intersection of practical ethics and theology, such as scholars in the interdisciplinary spaces of theological bioethics, Christian medical education, theological-philosophical ethics, and by ethics professionals who want to develop theologically rooted techniques in the midst of secularity. Because I specifically apply a theology of technique to clinical ethics consultation and give sustained attention to this application, it will be of special interest to Christian clinical ethicists and those in Christian healthcare contexts such as chaplains and mission and formation leaders. However, as we will see, liturgies are not just Christian activities but are human activities: we all engage in affective cultural rituals that form our desires and longings, and hence our character and our actions.[15] The liturgies we engage in our lives, whether secular or religious, form our moral sensibilities and help determine what we see (and don't see) when we are faced with moral questions. The kind of attention I devote to liturgy in the second part of this book is a uniquely Christian attention to a universal human phenomenon, and we all ought to interrogate the practices that influence our moral formation.

The Problem: Standardization of Clinical Ethics Techniques

How did we come to believe that standardized technique is essential for quality?[16] There are different possible answers to this question. The shift in all practical ethics disciplines from an emphasis on content to one on process has been well documented and discussed for at least forty years. I will offer Margaret Walker's telling of this shift, which is corroborated by the telling Jeffrey P. Bishop offers elsewhere twenty-three years later, among many others in between. Walker wrote in 1993 that "Literature of the last fifteen years on moral expertise and ethics consulting shows a shift in emphasis from issues of *content* to those of *process*—from what the ethicist knows, to what the ethicist does or enables."[17] On her account, this shift parallels two adjacent and concurrent shifts from "what" to "how:" (1) the institutionalization of hospital ethics committees after the Joint Commission requirement in 1992,[18] which reflects the need to demonstrate external (to the field) value, and (2) movements in philosophy and ethics to acknowledge situatedness and embeddedness in moral communities, which reflects an internal (to the field) shift.

These two moves were, of course, reactions to what had been going on before them. There was a sense that philosophy and ethics had become mainly about code-like moral systems that had little to no bearing on the "real world," especially in contexts as messy and dynamic as medicine. "General moral maxims or principles can often be connected to particular instances only by a thick tissue of perceptions and interpretations;" writes Walker, "these are fed by diverse skills and rooted in varied habits of thought and feeling. Moral competence is thus not reducible to a codelike decision instrument (much less an algorithmic one) any more than carpentry is reducible to a saw."[19] There was also an acknowledgment, in the vein of 1980s–1990s postmodern critique, that all of our moral systems are contingent upon cultural context. Moral sensibilities are embedded in a particular social setting and cannot be abstracted as "pure" moral truth. This means that even the doing of ethics is an element of culture building; we cannot have moral discourse that is immune from being changed as we engage it together. In essence, as Walker tells the story, with these related realizations it became necessary and right to critique prevailing static ways of conceiving of ethics and begin to acknowledge particularity and the flexibility of moral systems. Thus, an attention shift from *what* to *how*.

But these shifts were double-edged swords. What Walker (and a good many others) could not see in those early days is that valuable critiques were leading clinical ethicists to trade one kind of blunt standardization for another. Rather than standardized ethical *theories* that were inflexible to context, nuance, and particularity, the clinical ethicists of the early 1990s chose to begin standardizing *systems, methods, and processes* for the performance of clinical ethics that have, by now, become just as inflexible to nuance and particularity. As I will argue later, inflexibility is not an inevitable feature of practical ethics techniques; rather, inflexibility is a result of certain choices about the appropriate features of an ethics technique and, above all, their *standardization* across contexts. Early clinical ethicists' critiques were necessary and right; their next move simply shifted the problem—from standardization in what the ethicist *knows* or *believes* to standardization in what the ethicist *does*.[20] As I hope to show in the early pages of my project, this shift was (1) just as problematic for robust ethics, and (2) brought with it a host of problems (some old, some new) that we have not fully acknowledged or understood in the decades since.

Jeffrey P. Bishop offers a complementary telling of this shift in his 2017 article "Principles, Rules, and the Deflation of the Good in Bioethics."[21] In the early days of formal bioethics, in the wake of gross research ethics and human rights violations both domestically (i.e., Tuskegee) and abroad (i.e., Nazi Germany), philosophers were forced to articulate a set of norms and principles that could hold and be applied globally, across cultures. Just like in my evaluation of the shift from content to process, Bishop finds this well-intentioned move had unintended consequences. The move to generalized moral principles required a deflation of the metaphysical concepts that have always been at the heart of ethics, namely those of the good and of persons. In an attempt to evade relativism, to have something normative to say across cultures, metaphysics was sidelined and general mid-level principles were elevated. This led directly to an emphasis on *right action* rather than the concrete goods of persons because action can be policed while beliefs cannot. What Bishop concludes is similar to what I will argue in this book: "Because medicine is aimed at health, and the goods possible for persons in health, any ethics of medicine must be grounded in a philosophy of the goods for persons and goods of persons."[22] In other words, we have to get back to metaphysics if we are to do ethics.

Both Walker and Bishop seem to agree that modern ethics' shift to right action has been in some way a reaction to secularism and pluralism.[23] Clinical ethicists have always been grappling with how to establish ourselves in a world full of diverse metaphysical commitments.[24] In fact, there has been a robust record of this grappling in the literature, with bioethicists asking:

> How much of the traditional concerns of ethics for normative questions can survive? Can bioethics, in its present state, withstand the challenges of postmodernism without slipping into moral relativism, nihilism, or chaos? Can, or should, the foundations of ethics in moral philosophy be recovered, eliminated, or modified, and in what way?[25]

Walker and other practical ethicists in the latter half of the twentieth century were not wrong in their dissatisfaction with rigid moral systems and in their belief that those systems were failing us in practical settings. But when it comes to CEC, the most contextual and practical segment of bioethics, normativity amidst secularity cannot be secured by the implementation of standardized processes, principles, and techniques. In fact, the standardization approach puts practical ethics in even more grave peril. As I will argue in the pages to come, an ethics aimed at right action alone is no ethics at all.

Bioethicists around the turn of the century such as Ruth Macklin,[26] Tom Beauchamp,[27] H. Tristram Engelhardt,[28] Gilbert Meilaender,[29] and Alasdair MacIntyre[30] all noticed the erosion of *ethics* in bioethics. Each offers valuable suggestions for reclaiming normative footing. As Edmund Pellegrino says succinctly,

> In short, the first item on the agenda of the bioethicist for the next century will be to decide whether bioethics will be authentically an enterprise of ethics, or instead, it will become an amorphous expanding universe of preferences, opinions, feelings, or value choices filled with exquisite existential detail but enfeebled by a lack of normative content.[31]

But even Pellegrino fails to acknowledge that the problem is never just a lack of normative content—although that in itself is a problem in our postmodern climate. As we erode the *what* from clinical ethics, we are simultaneously strengthening the *how*: our processes and procedures are threatening to override moral seriousness and assert their place as the true content of clinical ethics. Ana Iltis identified this very thing in 2000:

> Because we have no universally agreed upon background moral theory which can serve as the basis for bioethical decision-making, [contemporary bioethicists] try to move bioethics away from theory. For them, a good method of bioethical decision-making is one which resolves cases in ways that are justifiable to the parties involved, not necessarily in ways that bring us "close" to the right and the true.[32]

Standardized processes and procedures in fact have normative pull away from robust moral inquiry aimed at the right and the true, as I aim to show in Part I.

What is more, standardized ethics techniques, like all techniques, arise out of fundamental commitments to a way of seeing the world. In other words, they enact certain ontologies. In this way they are like secular liturgies: rubrics for worship, attuning us to certain aspects of reality and concealing others.[33] The pertinent question is, then: to what do standardized CEC techniques attune us, and what do they teach us to "worship?" I will argue that standardized CEC techniques operate within a false ontology, a false conception of the nature of being, and thus constitute *ersatz* liturgies setting us up to "worship" the false gods of power, control, and progress.[34] I will fully flesh out this critique in Chapter 2 and offer Christian liturgical theology as a corrective in Part II.

To recognize when we have been caught up in problematic practices like these is not easy, especially given our intention to help those in distress, to see that the right thing is done, and to offer compassionate support to patients, families, and medical professionals. Yet recognize we must. Rowan Williams calls this the "difficult work" of ethics: discovering how one has been shaped and is being shaped for good or ill.[35] Every practical ethicist enters their career with good intentions. It will likely be difficult for ethicists to engage in the kind of self-critique I am encouraging; I know it is difficult for me. Yet, I hope to show that in our haste to standardize CEC techniques we may have inadvertently participated in the alienation of patients (as-persons) in medicine, subtly refusing to encounter them and behold them, to be human alongside and with them, to allow our vulnerabilities to surface, and to implicate ourselves in their good. In short, we have participated in a technocratic medicine. In equating ethics with standardized techniques we have been complicit in a refusal to be responsive and responsible, which are the bedrock of what it means to be an ethicist. We must reorient our practices in order to remain accountable to those we serve, and I believe learning from liturgical rubrics is the best place to start.

In sum, while the desire for reliable and high-quality CEC is a commendable one, I am convinced we cannot accomplish it by standardizing our ethics consultation method(s). To develop and implement the "right" technique(s) will only pull us further away from the free, rich, and full ethical inquiry that characterizes the best of CEC. While others have made similar claims before me, no one has fully identified the reasons why; as a result, dissenters to standardization are largely a sidelined group on the margins of bioethics. I aim to draw dissenters back into the conversation by engaging the deeper questions of metaphysics in CEC in a theologically and philosophically robust way, and ultimately to offer a rethinking of the theology of practical ethics.

Because techniques have become our flavor of standardization today, I will give sustained attention to five major CEC methods that are most commonly taught and practiced. I will then offer specific recommendations for new, nonstandardized, local CEC techniques, so that this project is practically applicable to those who are directly engaging ethical conflicts in medicine. What is at stake is no less than the very possibility of normative bioethics in the coming century.

Notes

1 "Color Blindness, History, and the Law" by Kimberlé Williams Crenshaw, copyright © 1997 by Kimberlé Williams Crenshaw; from THE HOUSE THAT RACE BUILT: BLACK AMERICANS, U.S. TERRAIN by Wahneema Lubiano. Used by permission of Pantheon Books, an imprint of the Knopf Doubleday Publishing Group, a division of Penguin Random House LLC. All rights reserved. Kimberle Williams Crenshaw, "Color Blindness, History, and the Law," in *The House That Race Built*, ed. Wahneema Lubiano (New York: Vintage Books, 2010; reprint, Kindle).

2 Stuart G. Finder and Mark J. Bliton, *Peer Review, Peer Education, and Modeling in the Practice of Clinical Ethics Consultation: The Zadeh Project* (Cham: Springer Open, 2018). This book is licensed under the terms of the Creative Commons Attribution 4.0 International License (http://creativecommons.org/licenses/by/4.0/). No changes were made.

3 In this book, I am discussing American bioethics only.

4 For some examples, see Jeffrey P. Bishop, Joseph B. Fanning, and Mark J. Bilton, "Of Goods and Goals and Floundering About: A Dissensus Report on Clinical Ethics Consultation," *HEC Forum* 21, no. 3 (2009): 275–91; G. R. Scofield, "Ethics Consultation: The Least Dangerous Profession?" *Cambridge Quarterly of Healthcare Ethics* 2, no. 4 (1993): 417–26; H. Tristram Engelhardt, "Credentialing Strategically Ambiguous and Heterogeneous Social Skills: The Emperor without Clothes," *HEC Forum*, no. 3 (2009): 293–306; Lisa M. Rasmussen, "Non-Certain Foundations: Clinical Ethics Consultation for the Rest of Us," in *At the Foundations of Bioethics and Biopolitics: Critical Essays on the Thought of H. Tristram Engelhardt, Jr.*, ed. Lisa M. Rasmussen, Ana Iltis, and Mark J. Cherry

(Cham: Springer International Publishing, 2015); Rasmussen, Iltis, and Cherry, *At the Foundations of Bioethics and Biopolitics*; A. Brummett and E. K. Salter, "Taxonomizing Views of Clinical Ethics Expertise," *American Journal of Bioethics* 19, no. 11 (2019): 50–61; Abram Brummett and Christopher J. Ostertag, "Two Troubling Trends in the Conversation over Whether Clinical Ethics Consultants Have Ethics Expertise," *HEC Forum* 30, no. 2 (2018): 157–69; David J. Casarett and Frona Daskal, "The Authority of the Clinical Ethicist," *Hastings Center Report* 28, no. 6 (1998): 6–11.

5 Analysis of the HEC-C exam and certification is ongoing. See Claire Horner et al., "What the Hec-C? An Analysis of the Healthcare Ethics Consultant-Certified Program: One Year In," *American Journal of Bioethics*, no. 3 (2020): 9–18; Julie Aultman and Cynthia Pathmathasan, "A Call for Diversity and Inclusivity in the Hec-C Program," *The American Journal of Bioethics* 20, no. 3 (2020): 46–50; James A. Hynds and Joseph A Raho, "A Profession without Expertise? Professionalization in Reverse," *The American Journal of Bioethics* 20, no. 3 (2020): 44–6.

6 Bishop, Fanning, and Bilton, "Of Goods and Goals and Floundering About: A Dissensus Report on Clinical Ethics Consultation."

7 Sharon L. Feldman et al., "Answering the Call for Standardized Reporting of Clinical Ethics Consultation," *Journal of Clinical Ethics* 31, no. 2 (Summer 2020): 173–7.

8 Douglas J. Opel et al., "Integrating Ethics and Patient Safety: The Role of Clinical Ethics Consultants in Quality Improvement," *The Journal of Clinical Ethics* 20, no. 3 (2009): 220–7.

9 Many have demonstrated as such: Jeffrey P. Bishop, Joseph B. Fanning, and Mark J. Bilton, "Echo Calling Narcissus: What Exceeds the Gaze of Clinical Ethics Consultation?" *HEC Forum* 22, no. 1 (2010): 73–84; Tristram Engelhardt, "Credentialing Strategically Ambiguous and Heterogeneous Social Skills: The Emperor without Clothes"; Annie Friedrich, "The Pitfalls of Proceduralism: An Exploration of the Goods Internal to the Practice of Clinical Ethics Consultation," *HEC Forum* 30, no. 4 (2018): 389–403.

10 Robert Orr and Wayne Shelton, "A Process and Format for Clinical Ethics Consultation," *The Journal of Clinical Ethics* 20, no. 1 (Spring 2009): 2. Italics added.

11 Nancy Dubler and Jeffrey Blustein, "Credentialing Ethics Consultants: An Invitation to Collaboration," *American Journal of Bioethics* 7, no. 2 (2007): 35.

12 Nicholas Yue Shuen Yoon et al., "Evaluating Assessment Tools of the Quality of Clinical Ethics Consultations: A Systematic Scoping Review from 1992 to 2019," *BMC Medical Ethics* 21, no. 1 (2020): 51. Italics added.

13 Opel et al., "Integrating Ethics and Patient Safety: The Role of Clinical Ethics Consultants in Quality Improvement," 222.

14 Dennis F. Thompson, "What Is Practical Ethics?," in *Ethics at Harvard 1907–2007*, ed. The President and Fellows of Harvard College (Harvard University Edmond J. Safra Foundation Center for Ethics, 2007).

15 James K. A. Smith, *You Are What You Love: The Spiritual Power of Habit* (Grand Rapids, MI: Brazos Press, 2016); *Desiring the Kingdom: Worship, Worldview, and Cultural Formation*, ed. James K. A. Smith, Cultural Liturgies (Grand Rapids, MI: Baker Academic, 2009).

16 It's hard to say exactly when we came to believe this; it was still up for debate at least in 2009, as evidenced by George Agich's article "Why Quality Is Addressed So Rarely in Clinical Ethics Consultation," *Cambridge Quarterly of Healthcare Ethics* 18, no. 4 (October 2009): 339–46, where he argues that quality must be assessed on a local level, from within the practice of CEC rather than on an institutional level, and that quality need not be reliant on standardized techniques.

17 Margaret Urban Walker, "Keeping Moral Space Open," *Hastings Center Report* 23, no. 2 (1993): 33–40. Italics added.

18 "Accreditation Manual for Hospitals," ed. Joint Commission on Accreditation of Health Care Organizations (Oakbrook Terrace, 1992).

19 Walker, "Keeping Moral Space Open," 34.

20 The elevation of pragmatic solutions that work and are useful, rather than what is true and good, is noted also by Ana Smith Iltis, "Bioethics as Methodological Case Resolution: Specification, Specified Principlism and Casuistry," *The Journal of Medicine and Philosophy* 25, no. 3 (2000): 271–84. Casarett and Daskal, "The Authority of the Clinical Ethicist," and Edmund D. Pellegrino, "Bioethics at Century's Turn: Can Normative Ethics Be Retrieved?," *Journal of Medicine & Philosophy* 25, no. 6 (2000): 656.

21 Jeffrey P. Bishop, "Principles, Rules, and the Deflation of the Good in Bioethics," *Ethics, Medicine, and Public Health* 3 (2017): 440–51.

22 Ibid., 445.

23 Edmund Pellegrino agrees in his insightful article: Pellegrino, "Bioethics at Century's Turn: Can Normative Ethics Be Retrieved?" The irony is that the

reaction against secularism has actually reified secularity in our ethics techniques and procedures. I will return to the idea that standardized CEC techniques are secular liturgies in Chapters 2 and 6.

24 Engelhardt, "Credentialing Strategically Ambiguous and Heterogeneous Social Skills: The Emperor without Clothes."
25 Pellegrino, "Bioethics at Century's Turn: Can Normative Ethics Be Retrieved?" 656.
26 Ruth Macklin, *Against Relativism: Cultural Diversity and the Search for Ethical Universals in Medicine* (Oxford: Oxford University Press, 1999).
27 Tom L. Beauchamp, "Reply to Strong on Principlism and Casuistry," *The Journal of Medicine and Philosophy* 25, no. 3 (2000): 342–7.
28 H. Tristram Engelhardt, Jr., *The Foundations of Bioethics*, 2nd ed. (Oxford: Oxford University Press, 1996).
29 Gilbert Meilaender, *Body, Soul, and Bioethics* (Notre Dame, IN: University of Notre Dame Press, 1995).
30 Alasdair C. MacIntyre, *Three Rival Versions of Moral Enquiry: Encyclopaedia, Genealogy, and Tradition: Being Gifford Lectures Delivered in the University of Edinburgh in 1988* (Notre Dame, IN: University of Notre Dame Press, 1990).
31 Pellegrino, "Bioethics at Century's Turn: Can Normative Ethics Be Retrieved?" 661.
32 Iltis was specifically referring to the authors in the June 2000 issue of the *Journal of Medicine and Philosophy*, which include the mainstream figures Albert Jonsen, Tom Beauchamp, Carson Strong, Bernard Gert, Charles Culver, Danner Clouser, and Henry Richardson. See Iltis, "Bioethics as Methodological Case Resolution: Specification, Specified Principlism and Casuistry."
33 For a development of "secular liturgies," see especially chapter 3 of James K. A. Smith, *Imagining the Kingdom: How Worship Works*, ed. James K. A. Smith, Cultural Liturgies (Grand Rapids, MI: Baker Academic, 2013).; See also *Desiring the Kingdom: Worship, Worldview, and Cultural Formation*.
34 There is precedent for identifying secular *ersatz* liturgies in medicine. Building from sources like Catherine Pickstock and James K. A. Smith, Jeffrey P. Bishop and Kimbell Kornu argue that certain practices of modern medicine are *ersatz* liturgies worshipping false gods and orienting participants around their worship. See Jeffrey P. Bishop, "Of Idolatries and Ersatz Liturgies: The False Gods of Spiritual Assessment," *Christian Bioethics* 19, no. 3 (2013): 332–47; Kimbell

Kornu, "Medical Ersatz Liturgies of Death: Anatomical Dissection and Organ Donation as Biopolitical Practices," *Heythrop Journal* 63, no. 3 (2020): 386–400.

35 Rowan Williams, "On Making Moral Decisions," *Anglican Theological Review* 81, no. 2 (Spring 1999): 295–308.

Part I

Standardized Clinical Ethics Consultation Techniques

1

What Is a Technique?

Men have become the tools of their tools. —Henry David Thoreau[1]

The first task in my critique of practical ethics techniques is to explain what I mean by "technique"—surely we cannot critique (or indeed, rebuild) something without knowing what it is and what it is for.[2] In the case of technique, as with most things, the deeper one goes into the question "what is it?" the harder it is to answer. A simple definition such as "a method for doing something" obscures the deeper meaning of technique and limits our moral imagination. It is more helpful to zoom out and locate techniques within a broader discourse. The philosopher Martin Heidegger considers technique a type of technology, in the broader category of *techne* (Greek for technique or technology). While it may seem odd, because we tend to think of technology only as devices, widening our view to this broader category helps make space for a fresh line of critique regarding techniques in practical ethics. After exploring Heidegger's thoughts on what exactly *techne* is, I will locate standardized CEC methods within his framework, identifying them as a type of *techne* that is insufficient for ethics. Finally, I will identify parallel lines of thought in a few other philosophers. These lines of thought will re-emerge, weaving in and out of the rest of this book.

Heidegger on *Techne*

Heidegger, in his seminal essay "The Question Concerning Technology," identifies the question "what is it?" as (you guessed it) *the* central question concerning technology. But rather than offering a precise or narrow definition, such as Grant's "the whole apparatus of instruments made by man and placed at the disposal of man for his choices and purposes,"[3] Heidegger turns the tables and argues that such definitions merely reinforce an instrumental understanding of technology—the belief that technology merely consists of instruments and tools that can be put to whatever use we desire. And if we understand technology instrumentally, we fail to understand the ways technology functions in the human lifeworld and the ways it influences us.

Instrumental definitions, writes Heidegger, beg the question. If we were to gather up all the objects we typically call "technology" and attempt to define their commonalities, we would be no closer to understanding the "what-is-it?" of technology than before. Rather, we would reinforce our preconceptions about what technology is by examining only those objects we already define as technologies. So long as we perpetuate our preconceptions and go no deeper, "we remain unfree and chained to technology,"[4] says Heidegger, because we fail to interrogate the *essence* of technology, which is an ontological endeavor. Said another way, "what is it?" is not a question of linguistic or practical definition, but a question of metaphysics.

Having rejected instrumental definitions of technology, Heidegger writes that *techne* is the name for the activities and skills of the craftsman, the arts of the mind, and the fine arts. Notice he does not equate *techne* with devices. Less satisfying than precise definitions, perhaps, yet this framing opens a different world of possible inquiry. For one, it shows that techniques are technologies. The embodied and applied skill of makers, thinkers, and artists is just as much a part of *techne* as are the physical tools they use to carry out their making and thinking. Techniques and technologies have the same character, the same essence; they are of one mind. We can assess the work of technique as we assess the work of technology.

This is the first of four key concepts from "The Question Concerning Technology" that are foundational for an analysis of CEC methods. In brief: (1) *Techne* includes both technology and technique, and thus the philosophy of technology applies equally to both, (2) *Techne* is not a thing (object or process) but a mode of revealing, (3) *Techne* is thus never neutral, and (4) *Techne* can operate in two ways: bringing-forth (*poiesis*) or challenging-forth. These four ideas have direct import for how we understand CEC techniques.

First, Heidegger's locating of both technology and technique within the category of *techne* means that we can extend the discourse on the philosophy of technology to interrogate technique as well. To begin here sets us on a path that already diverges from most analyses of technique, which assume that techniques are neutral tools to achieve whatever ends we desire (the instrumental understanding). Again—in the case of all *techne*—instrumental definitions beg the question concerning ontology and blind us to the powerful formative work techniques bring to bear on us, their users. There is something deeper at work in technique as a form of *techne*, and philosophers of technology help us to examine practical ethics techniques on the metaphysical level.

Next, having acknowledged that the activities, skills, and objects of *techne* are more than their instrumental or anthropological functions, Heidegger finally attends to the ontological question. He writes that *techne* is not merely a thing or a process but a *mode of revealing*. "[*Techne*] reveals whatever does not bring itself forth and does not yet lie here before us."[5] So long as we regard *techne* merely instrumentally, as means to an end (although modes of revealing are at least those things), we "grasp something that is correct, and yet never touch its nature, which is a producing that brings something forth," makes something present, allows something to appear.[6]

Techne thus refers not to individual objects like iPhones and MRI scanners or even individual activities like driving a car, but rather modes of revealing, or ways of seeing. Modes of revealing form our gaze and determine our field of perception, allowing certain things to come into relief for us. Modes of revealing are thus world-creators; they are ways of constructing, delimiting, and molding the multiplicitous realities before us to appear one way and not a million possible others. The oft-quoted truism comes to mind: to the person with a hammer, everything looks like a nail. Ontologically, *techne* is the thing that makes human doing and making possible by revealing to us a world that can be known, used, and ordered. *Techne* is the thing that permits certain elements of reality to come into view. Another way of putting it is that *techne* is doing work for us, but not only the work we think it's doing. The instrumental understanding of *techne* is not incorrect—*techne* always has an instrumental function—but the kind of work *techne* is doing is *on ourselves* as much as on the world around us.[7]

This understanding leads to the third key concept: as a way of seeing, *techne* is never neutral, as we so commonly imagine technology/technique to be. Rather, *techne* already sets us on a moral pursuit by virtue of determining what we notice and how it appears. Thus, *techne* can be referred to as a modern "cultural imaginary" in the sense that Charles Taylor understands it.[8] We cannot say that our techniques are merely tools to be freely used toward whatever ends we intend. It is more accurate to say that the techniques we employ actually shape and determine the ends we intend. *Techne* is a mode of revealing that we use or practice to construct a world. In so doing, we define and delineate our own place and intention in that world. Thus, the being of technique and the being that technique permits to come into view for its user are interconnected.

Lastly for our purposes, Heidegger delineates between two ways *techne* can reveal. It can reveal through bringing-forth (*poiesis*), or through challenging-forth. *Techne* historically belonged only to the former, the realm of bringing-forth, which it did via the techniques and skills of craftsmanship, intelligence, and the fine arts. *Techne* was, and is, a collection of pursuits aimed at unconcealing, uncovering, allowing to behold, something true about the world that is not immediately obvious. The practice of CEC should properly fall into this category; it is a collection of pursuits aimed at unconcealing what is good in a particular context for particular persons. In contrast, says Heidegger, our modern technologies and modern techniques of ordering are a new and different kind of *techne*.[9] Modern *techne* aims to uncover not through *poiesis*, but through challenging-forth, an unlocking and exposing of resources for extraction and storage, and it aims to use those resources toward ends external to the source.[10] When standardized CEC techniques aim to mediate or resolve moral conflicts in a reliable and repeatable way, they are in fact challenging-forth, delimiting the types of results that can emerge and requiring that a result does emerge so that work can go on. Unlike *poiesis*, challenging-forth is not responsive to the unique qualities of the objects it reveals. Rather, it acts universally. In other words—it is standardized.

Challenging-forth is a mode that constrains our gaze, making possible certain lines of inquiry. Techniques allow a certain world to come into relief for their users—or certain features of the world, which the user then comes to equate with the world itself. In the type of technique that challenges-forth, we are trained to see being as a "calculable complex of the effects of forces,"[11] which does uncover certain types of truth about the world. Challenging-forth is quite naturally at home in modern science and medicine: "Thus when man, investigating, observing, pursues nature as an area of his own conceiving, he has already been claimed by a way of revealing that challenges him to approach nature *as an object of research . . .*"[12] So challenging-forth is quite effective and appropriate for systematically investigating objects of research. It is effective and appropriate for medical professionals to operate mainly in this mode because it allows them to make sense of disparate facts, symptoms, reactions, etc., and treat their patients according to medical standards of care. In fact, as we take up with challenging-forth, it makes sure we see the world in a way that enables ordering. It moves us toward efficiency, efficacy, and repeatability in our scientific and medical pursuits.[13] So, "[challenging-forth] can indeed permit correct determinations; but precisely through these successes the danger may remain that in the midst of all that is correct the true will withdraw," as Heidegger says.[14] It enables us, but in its enabling, challenging-forth limits us in other ways; it does not allow for a free and full encounter with *the ontological essence of what is unconcealed*. Because rather than allowing for an encounter with essence, which is messy and dynamic and which contains multitudes, challenging-forth enables reliable usage and effectiveness by allowing only those features of reality which can be manipulated to emerge. Like all techniques, those operating in the mode of challenging-forth reveal a world to us; but they do not allow us to behold the world. As I will argue in Chapter 2, challenging-forth conceals the very elements of the world that make ethical engagement possible.

Heidegger's *Techne* within the Philosophy of Technology

Philosophers of technology before and after Heidegger have answered our original question "what is it?" in slightly different ways. Yet they share at least two important themes that are worth drawing out before we turn our attention back to CEC methods. First, humanity and *techne* are inherently interconnected, and second, *techne* is a necessary element of human being and becoming. We cannot do away with techniques wholesale, but we also cannot afford to adopt them without critical engagement and awareness of their effect on us and on our perception.

One of the earliest philosophers of technology, Ernst Kapp (1808–96), writes that human organs and body parts were the initial blueprints for tools, machines, and even entire cultural systems.[15] Because humans relate to the world through our bodily organs, Kapp writes, we come to see the world outside of us as organ-like as well. "Unconsciously, the finger is projected into the stylus, the arm into the axe, and the nervous system into the telegraphic network, allowing humans to emerge as cultural beings—that is to say, to emerge at all."[16] Our bodies, then, constrain our gaze such that what we see when we look at a stick may be not just a stick, but a potential extension of our fingers.

Subsequently, the tools/technologies/techniques we create reflexively form *us* when we use them. The idea that our tools create us after we create them leads Kapp to offer a theory of "culture as technologically conditioned, as *operation*."[17] In other words, human culture is created through the deployment of technologies. Projecting their organs outward onto technological objects (i.e., using a stylus as an extension of the finger), humans then come to learn about their own body and mind through the lens of the tool, in a dialectical process.[18] Culture is built upon and around these understandings that the human comes to belatedly, as a result of technology use. Human bodies, human culture, and the tools/technologies/techniques we use are thus intricately intertwined, even inseparable. Human being and becoming are tied up with the technological. Thus, Kapp is able to lay the foundation for later philosophers of technology to find no distinct dichotomy between subject and object, human and tool.[19] While humans project their organs onto the objects they use, it is the operation of those technologies that makes the human form comprehensible to the human.[20] Kapp establishes an inseparability, then, of use and being.[21] The connection between technology use and human being means, of course, that the creation and use of *techne* (*technik*, in German) actually allowed for the emergence of human beings as such and the development of human culture. This line of thinking allows for the later development of theories of *kulturtechnik* (cultural techniques), which assert that operation and being are closely entangled in human culture.[22]

Cultural historian and philosopher Walter Ong (1912–2003) agrees with Kapp that technology and human being have a dialectical relationship.[23] The tools we use and the culture we create influence our perception of the world, and vice versa. In his seminal book *Orality and Literacy*, Ong posits that the shift in (most) human cultures from orality to literacy—a technological change—brings about a fundamental change in worldview within those cultures.[24] For Ong, this change is tinged with loss; he laments the shift from the world of sound to the world of sight, from what he identifies as a basic openness and receptivity toward the world around us (typified by the ear) to an "objective" gaze peering out at the world around us (typified by the eye). The development of the techniques of writing and reading, says Ong, shifted human perception so much that culture was fundamentally changed, and the modern era was allowed to emerge. "Without writing, the literate mind would not and could not think as it does, not only when engaged in writing but normally even when it is composing its thoughts in oral form. More than any other single invention, writing has transformed human consciousness."[25] Both Kapp's and Ong's theses are consistent with Heidegger's: technology is not neutral, and utility on its own cannot get at what really matters when evaluating technology, which is the moral bearing of technology on human perception and human life.

Peter-Paul Verbeek is one of the most important voices interrogating the moral bearing of technology on human life. Taking a narrower definition of technology than Kapp and Ong—Verbeek attends principally to devices—he rejects the popular idea that a moral subject charges an object with moral value when the subject picks up the tool.[26] In other words, in keeping with other philosophers of technology, Verbeek rejects the instrumental definition of technology that assumes moral neutrality. Rather, he argues, some form of agency is built into the tool from the very beginning. Verbeek argues that the user is decentralized from the start because the technology has already begun to alter the subject's intentionality; it has its own built-in tendencies. If we take Heidegger to be correct that technique has the same character as technology, then technique also has its own built-in tendencies. *Techne* is not a neutral tool; rather, it is endowed with certain tendencies, and it mediates our perception of the world in prescribed ways.[27] Moral evaluation of *techne* thus cannot focus on utility—"does it work?" —because utility assumes that subjects have full control and mastery over their *techne* and denies *techne's* reciprocal work on subjects.

French philosopher Jacques Ellul, more than any other, is directly critical of standardized technique. In fact, he claims that the situation is even worse than the preceding scholars believe. It is not just that *techne* is morally weighted; for Ellul, the dominance of standardized technique *in particular* makes it impossible to reach moral judgments through them.[28] In his book *The Technological Society*, Ellul reverses the often-assumed "hierarchy" of *techne*: rather than machines being the most obvious and primary manifestation of *techne*, and techniques being related to their use, Ellul writes that technique is primary, and machines are the "most obvious, massive, and impressive example *of technique*."[29] Standardized technique (and Ellul is thinking only of standardized technique, not a technique in the mode of *poiesis*) is in fact the primary manifestation of the technological, and machines are entirely dependent upon it:

> Technique integrates the machine into society. It constructs the kind of world the machine needs and introduces order where the incoherent banging of machinery heaped up ruins. It clarifies, arranges, and rationalizes; it does in the domain of the abstract what the machine did in the domain of labor. It is efficient and brings efficiency to everything.[30]

The primacy of attention that Ellul gives to technique as a form—really, *the* form—of *techne* is quite unique in the philosophical literature. While his outlook may be considered excessively bleak, Ellul offers valuable precedent for extending Heideggerian critique to standardized technique, not as an afterthought but as a primary consideration. Widely considered his most important book, *The Technological Society* is one of the most forceful and comprehensive social philosophies of technological civilization that has been written.[31]

Ellul's main concern is that the logic of technique is overriding the human. The most dangerous aspect of technique, he writes, is that it uses the human for the purposes of the machine. When standardized technique enters into human domains,[32] it uses for its medium the very substance of the human body, progressively absorbing it and integrating into it the values of the technological. Like Kapp and Ong, as well as Verbeek, Ellul acknowledges the power of *techne* to reshape human biology, psychology, and then culture. But beyond others, Ellul is profoundly pessimistic about the effects of standardized technique on humanity. He laments "the way in which [technique] is in process of taking over the traditional values of every society without exception, subverting and suppressing these values to produce at last a monolithic world culture in which all nontechnological difference and variety is mere appearance."[33] Our progressively technological civilization is "committed to the quest for continually improved means to carelessly examined ends."[34] Ellul is concerned that our fixation on process and procedure turns ends into means, and means into ends—"'know-how' takes on an ultimate value."[35] Rather than scholars and professionals in various fields, we increasingly have only technicians who compare rival techniques, judged in terms of "what is useful rather than what is good. Purposes drop out of sight and efficiency becomes the central concern."[36] It seems that standardization, for Ellul, is exactly what divides technique from other types of action, which have spontaneity as their essential character.

What exactly does he mean by standardization of technique, and what does he understand to be the danger? Ellul takes as authoritative Antoine Mas's definition:

> Standardization means resolving *in advance* all the problems that might possibly impede the functioning of an organization. It is not a matter of leaving it to inspiration, or ingenuity, nor even intelligence to find a solution at the moment some difficulty arises; it is rather in some way to anticipate both the difficulty and its resolution. From then on, standardization creates *impersonality*, in the sense that organization [sic] relies more on methods and instructions than on individuals.[37]

Standardized technique glosses over human being, "smothers the ideas that put its rule in question," and allows into public discourse only those ideas which already agree with the values of the technique.[38]

The effects of standardized action, as observed by Ellul, include increased efficiency, loss of locality and contextuality, loss of diversity, impossibility of aesthetic considerations, and reduced freedom for practitioners to choose between possible means.[39] Certainly in clinical ethics, these effects represent significant costs. While they enable us to reach certain goals, such as faster resolution and higher consult volume, professional status, demonstrated institutional value, cost savings, and reduced risk of catastrophic violations by rogue ethicists, standardized technique means we are turned into a kind of technician. Variability is eliminated in favor of efficiency. As Catherine Pickstock observes, "it seems . . . that the modern bureaucratic world no longer receives one in person by offering to one a virtuous and honorable role which one could fill non-identically, according to one's native genius, but rather demands that one suppress this in order to become a mere cog in a machine."[40]

Thus we have arrived at one final point in Ellul's work that ethicists must acknowledge: following Andre Leroi-Gourhan, Ellul argues that technique is a "cloak for man, a kind of cosmic vestment" or "intermediary agency" between ourselves and a chaotic outer world.[41] Because technique depersonalizes us (technicians are always replaceable), it protects us from the vulnerability that personalization carries. Technique serves to both defend us from chaos and turn our adversaries (environmental, material, or living) into allies. This observation highlights the quasi-liturgical character of technique, to which we will return in coming chapters. Ellul's observation also highlights one of the benefits of standardized technique unrelated to professional standing, which is self-protection. If we are to resist standardized methods in CEC, we must acknowledge self-protection as one of the hidden motivations behind them and prepare to respond to the vulnerability that comes in their absence.

While Ellul is less optimistic than I am about the possibility for resistance, he considers bearing witness to the technological society the most revolutionary of all possible acts.[42] "His concept of the duty of a Christian, who stands uniquely (is 'present') at the point of intersection of this material world and the eternal world to come, is not to concoct ambiguous ethical schemes or programs of social action, but to testify to the truth of both worlds and thereby to affirm his freedom through the revolutionary nature of his religion."[43] In Part II, I will further explore these possibilities from the perspective of Christian theology.

Techno-Ontology: Challenging-Forth in Clinical Ethics Consultation

So techniques are a kind of *techne*, which means that ontologically, they are modes of revealing which humans enlist to construct the world around them.[44] This construction or revealing also implies a concealing, since some aspects of reality must fade into the background as others come front and center. Yet the revealing and concealing permitted by our techniques is not only one-way; techniques end up forming us into certain kinds of people as we use them, often in ways that we do not entirely intend. A thorough analysis of technique will require us to explore what is revealed *and* what is concealed, what world is created *and* what parts of reality are dismissed, as well as the effects of it all on us who use such techniques.

I have noted that Heidegger delineates two kinds of *techne*, and thus two kinds of technique: bringing-forth and challenging-forth. I have noted also that standardized CEC techniques challenge-forth rather than bring-forth. It's worth looking a little deeper at this claim. The key word here is *standardized*; while there are certain "*poiesis*-like" elements built into some CEC techniques, to the extent they are standardized, they are functioning in the mode of challenging-forth—and as Heidegger warns us, "where this ordering holds sway, it drives out every other possibility of revealing."[45] In other words, the act of standardizing locates techniques within the mode of challenging-forth, which is totalizing within its sphere. Challenging-forth will rule out the possibility of "*poiesis*-like" elements holding sway in CEC, even if they seem to be incorporated into the method used. The concept of totalization (whether challenging-forth can exist alongside *poiesis*, and whether *poiesis* can exist within structures that operate in the mode of challenging-forth) will re-emerge in the coming chapters as we turn to the specific methods.

For now: why does standardization automatically locate techniques within the mode of challenging-forth? The answer is quite simple. Standardized techniques of whatever sort are intended to function exactly the same way each time we use them, and they assume reliability and efficacy. Efficient[46] techniques, even if the user is unconscious of it, downplay features of particularity or dissent that would render the techniques ineffective. Users see only the features of reality that their procedures are set up to reveal. As Heidegger says, challenging-forth "can only enact its own groundless metaphysical assumptions by increasingly quantifying the qualitative ... and by leveling down all attempts to justify human meaning to empty optimization imperatives ... "[47] Our standardized CEC techniques ask that we form ethical inquiry into the image of static forms and formulas which are by definition universally applied. Standardized CEC methods replace prudential intuition with procedures, causing a mechanical performance, a "reign of the copy,"[48] to use Catherine Pickstock's language, to which I will return in Chapter 2. The world these techniques permit to emerge is one of predictability and universality, a world that can be efficiently managed.

Theological ethicist Ashley John Moyse makes a similar point in his book *Reading Karl Barth, Interrupting Moral Technique, Transforming Biomedical Ethics*. In his words:

> The illusion of efficient methodology, which moral techniques introduce, directs individuals toward . . . setting humans free from otherwise intractable dilemmas. These moral techniques erect various methods that orient the relative group of interested moral strangers within a grammatical systematic and make essential, namely, common, certain modes of speech and reasoning, while discounting and discouraging the particular.[49]

While Moyse is not focused specifically on their standardization, he sees in CEC methods the goal of efficiency: to bring the chaos of conflict with moral strangers[50] into a coherent and workable form for CECs. These moral techniques represent the fundamental position toward being that is characteristic of modern *techne*, or challenging-forth: all things can be ordered by the system. In keeping with Heidegger's idea that *techne* enacts metaphysical assumptions that frame our perception of being, Moyse prefers to refer to technology and technique as *techno-ontology* and thus escape the instrumental understanding:

> The *idea* of techno-ontology—technology as not merely a concept or construction but a way of seeing or a determining of our way of seeing the world—can therefore include a compendium of industrial, political, economic, and moral machinery that instrumentalizes knowing for the purposes of doing, and bureaucratizes both the control and the management

of persons surveyed by the panoptic gaze and corresponding judgement of technique.[51]

It may sound quite strong, especially when we have much better intentions. But a main goal of standardized CEC methods seems to be to efficiently navigate conflicts, to put in order the chaos of competing voices that would otherwise derail the medical system in which we operate. When the technique is completed, the ethical conflict is considered solved, merely because the process of the method has been implemented. In other words, the technique legitimizes the outcome. We put our trust in the apparatus; all the while, dissenting voices may be coated in a thin veneer of consensus, and the uniqueness of the situation and of the patient and family in front of us is pulled into form. The ethicist is ultimately concealed, too, behind methods and principles, and she becomes little more than her doing, her controlling, her carrying out of duty.[52] I suspect that even the ethicist, in using standardized methods, will eventually feel like a cog. While it may lend us a certain degree of psychological safety from the turmoil of personal agency within moral conflict, the price paid is quite high. We might feel that our jobs and our feelings are protected because we have followed the protocol, but we lose a great deal of moral agency as well.

As a result, all those gathered for CEC are subjected to the authority of systems, rather than to the call of those before us. Concrete "I"s and "Thou"s, to take up Martin Buber's language, become simply "we."[53] Like evidence-based medicine, repeatable methods of canonical morality are an expression of the average, not the concrete.[54] They abstract us from the actual; they enact an ethics of "endless repetition and standardized monotony,"[55] an ethics of efficient and efficacious procedure. This abandonment of the concrete is ironic because, as I chronicled in the Prelude, the impetus for the creation of standardized CEC techniques was a desire to step away from ethical theories that were inflexible to context, nuance, and particularity. Early clinical ethicists began to standardize systems and processes for clinical ethics, rather than theories, in an effort to attend to the concrete and the actual. What they failed to see is that inflexibility is an inevitable result of standardization, so they merely shifted the problem—from abstraction in the *what* to abstraction in the *how*. What we have now are techniques and procedures which, by definition, cannot attend to the concrete and the actual.

As we start off on a way of challenging-forth, ordering the actual as an object of research and quality improvement, we are in danger of, as Heidegger says,

> pursuing and promulgating nothing but what is revealed in ordering, and of deriving all [our] standards on this basis. Through this the other possibility is blocked—that [we] might rather be admitted sooner and ever more primally to the essence of what is unconcealed and to its unconcealment, in order that [we] might experience as [our] essence the requisite belonging to revealing.[56]

In other words, standardized techniques bring into relief a small sliver of reality, elements that fit coherently into a world of order and repetition, but reality far exceeds this sliver. While challenging-forth holds sway, the kind of revealing that is an ordering, other modes of revealing are impossible. We foreclose on openness to something new and unexpected. We foreclose on beholding the being of another person. When Heidegger says, "in the midst of all that is correct the true will withdraw,"[57] he means that a technically correct result may hide the truth of being. To behold the being of the other—a being that is non-identically repeated in each new moment—is to sense something true.[58] And as I will elaborate in the next chapter, openness to the being of the other is absolutely essential to ethical inquiry. In sum, standardized CEC techniques so constrain moral inquiry as to render it ineffective. Additionally, they constrain our gaze toward the efficient resolution of conflict and turn us into the kinds of people who will be increasingly incapable of tolerating significant difference, diversity, and disagreement in clinical settings.

But although the foregoing critique is forceful (I believe, justifiably so), I want to be careful to say two things: (1) clinical ethicists do not intentionally use standardized methods to treat everyone the same. Clinical ethicists know better than anyone that the exact features of each ethics consult are unique. CEC methods have mechanisms for noting these differences. Indeed, it may even seem like using standardized methods is a responsible way to conduct consults, given how complex, variable, and unstable situations of ethical conflict or uncertainty often are. Some methods, like Richard Zaner's Phenomenological Method, have even been developed to intentionally incorporate elements that look like *poiesis*, such as active listening, attending to reality, bracketing predetermined principles, etc. Additionally, (2) many or most clinical ethicists (there is not enough data to be precise) do not yet use a standardized method, but have developed their own flexible procedure(s) using a hybrid model. Alternatively, since most clinical ethicists (again, there is a lack of data on this) are aware of the multiple methods currently available, some may fluidly choose between them in responding to the contextuality of a case as it presents itself.[59] However, the foregoing critiques are actually *even more* critical given these two conditions. Let me explain why this is the case.

In response to (1) The possible unintentionality of challenging-forth on the part of clinical ethicists means that we need this type of critique all the more urgently. In fact, clinical ethicists are likely to be quite interested in it for precisely this reason: we want to embody responsible, responsive, and ethical methods for conducting CEC. Now is the time to consider what those might be before ASBH solidifies their *recommended* standardized approach into a directive.[60] While I worry that some CECs and administrators want CEC to operate in the mode of challenging-forth (i.e., for job security, financial incentives, hospital revenue, easier and quicker solutions to conflicts, lower lengths of stay, etc.), even if no one wanted CEC to operate in the mode of challenging-forth, it does when performed under a standardized method. Challenging-forth is totalizing within its sphere and rules out the possibility of *poiesis* holding sway, *even if* the method seems to incorporate some of its elements. The fact that some methods are made to look like bringing-forth only makes standardization and its attendant features more subtle.

In response to (2) Because all standardized models fall short of enabling moral inquiry, a combination of models will also fall short. Techniques constrain the gaze of their users, and standardized techniques do so in a mode of challenging-forth; a hybrid model that utilizes multiple standardized techniques will thus constrain in a hybrid variety of ways. Choosing between standardized methods does not solve the problem created by challenging-forth, because we are not escaping the *enframing* that each of these standardized techniques brings once they are begun. For Heidegger, *enframing* refers to the "frame" by which we engage reality around us, and in which things must appear according to the conditions of our historical moment and what our historical moment holds to be important. In other words, the way we see the world is conscribed by the frame, or *enframing*, of our historical context, typified in our tools and techniques. Remember, techniques are technical (*techne*-ical) and constructive devices designed to bring a certain world into relief, devices which then reflexively form their users. The pertinent question, then, at least for practical ethics, is what type of world is created or revealed by our techniques? And what type of people do we become in the process?

A narrative example may help show what is lost when we attend primarily to preformed concepts and to challenging-forth solutions rather than the fullness of a moral question. Attending physician Brent R. Carr relates his experience receiving an ethics consultation in a tragic case of a patient with treatment-refractory depression with anxious distress.[61] He describes the medical team's moral disquiet: apprehension and confusion regarding whether the patient should receive electroconvulsive therapy (ECT), a risky procedure for this patient given her clinical particularities. Dr. Carr writes,

> As the attending who was to perform the procedure, I felt it important these hesitations were at least discussed, if not resolved. As such, I suggested that the psychiatry team consider an ethics consultation, as this may offer some assistance and help deliberate over the emerging mixed emotions surrounding the case . . . The ethics consult would promote further discussion about these challenges and, hopefully, foster stronger team cohesiveness. (. . .)[62]

Dr. Carr next recounts his experience receiving the ethics recommendations in the chart, and his disappointment that they seemed to have overlooked his deeper moral concern, which had to do with the philosophical questions brewing beneath the surface for the medical team:

> Forty-eight hours later, I was asked to proceed with ECT. The resident reported the Ethics Consult was on the chart. It was a succinct summary that stated all the necessary legal obligations had been met, the established lack of capacity had been appropriately documented, attempts to "avoid harm" were present, and affirmed husband was legally able to consent . . . Brief, simple. Oddly, all team members and students now verbalized how comfortable they were with proceeding with ECT. All hesitation or concern had fully and immediately dissolved after this perfunctory consultation. I attempted to process with the residents and students why there was such an immediate resolution to their concerns. But I was met with silence.

> My first inclination was the feeling of disappointment, which I had inappropriately and initially attributed to the brevity of the consultation. It had responded to what was asked of it. Perhaps it was my disappointment in the trainees' seeming disinterest or unwillingness to absorb themselves into a philosophical endeavor. Or was this a displacement of my failure to engage our students and residents in an ethical debate? Was this simply the sequelae of the time constraints of a hectic service? The ethics consult seemed depreciated somehow—relegated as though it were a solitary lab order that had returned a simple, concrete value. And that was the end of the discussion and concerns.[63]

The ethics consultation had been reliably and efficiently completed, had taken into account the relevant legal and ethical concepts, and had issued defensible recommendations. The medical team was even sufficiently reassured by the process and chart note, their concerns evaporated, *and still the attending physician sensed something had been lost.* He goes on to write, "The deference to the Ethics Consultation as a finality felt more paternalistic than collaborative."[64] The decision to move forward with ECT, a decision that initially drew out the medical practitioners' moral concern and deep philosophical uncertainty as to the proper aims of medicine and its tolerable risks, became "more palatable" after ethics consultation.[65] The technically right decision may have been reached (we don't know based only on the narrative), but the opportunity for moral dialogue and rich conscientious engagement with reality had been squandered.

We do not know what method or technique was employed by the ethics consultant(s) who responded to Dr. Carr's consultation request. But we can tell based on the resulting product, the chart note, that the ethicist(s) attended to legal obligations, capacity, harm, and consent, yet missed the full color of the physician's moral concerns. We may draw the conclusion that their method was set up to reveal only such categories as are traditionally defined as "clinical ethics" (capacity, harm, consent, risk/benefit, etc.) but not to reveal the medical team's disquiet or Dr. Carr's hunger for robust exploration of values and duties. It is, of course, always possible that ethicists will miss important features of a case; yet how we design our methods will almost certainly affect the frequency of such errors.

So we return to the questions: what type of (moral) world is created or revealed by our techniques? And what type of people do we (and others) become in the process? Even those ethicists who refuse established techniques altogether and create their own processes should attend to these crucial questions. We should not eschew standardized methods on a contingent basis (i.e., until a "better" or "best" model is created). We should reject standardized methods on principled grounds, grounds that are articulated well enough to push back against ASBH's increasing process expectations. And we should be able to defend the non-standardized techniques we develop instead (more on this in the Interlude and Part II).

So standardized methods challenge-forth rather than bring-forth, because standardization itself—regardless of content—does not allow for *poiesis*. But some readers may still ask, "So our methods challenge-forth rather than bring-forth . . . so what? Don't they still work?" Thus I suspect more work remains to be done to convince readers that challenging-forth is, in fact, incompatible with robust ethics and that *poiesis* is the only appropriate mode. In the next chapter, I will show that standardized techniques won't work for practical ethics because the ontology revealed through challenging-forth is *fundamentally at odds* with the ontological essence of human being(s). And since practical ethics is a search for the good of being(s), we must at least have access to being(s) as a necessary precondition.

Notes

1 Henry David Thoreau, *Walden* (Boston, MA: Ticknor and Fields, 1854), https://archive.org/details/waldenorlifei00thor/page/40/mode/2up?q=%22their+tools%22.
2 This section of the book is based on earlier research that is published in HEC Forum. See Jordan Mason, "Techniques of Ordering and the Dynamism of Being," *HEC Forum* 35 (2022): 253-69.
3 George Grant, "Technology and Justice," in *Collected Works of George Grant*, ed. Arthur Davis and Henry Roper (Toronto: University of Toronto Press, 2009), 595.
4 Martin Heidegger, "The Question Concerning Technology," in *Basic Writings* (New York: HarperCollins Publishers, 1993), 311.

5 Ibid., 319.
6 Martin Heidegger, "Building Dwelling Thinking," in *Poetry, Language, Thought* (New York: Harper Colophon Books, 1971).
7 Peter-Paul Verbeek, "Obstetric Ultrasound and the Technological Mediation of Morality: A Postphenomenological Analysis," *Human Studies* 31, no. 1 (2008): 11–26; *Moralizing Technology: Understanding and Designing the Morality of Things* (Chicago, IL: University of Chicago Press, 2011).
8 Charles Taylor, *A Secular Age* (Cambridge: Belknap Press, 2007). Jeffrey Bishop refers to the *technological imaginary* as a cultural imaginary in his work. See Jeffrey P Bishop, "Ageing and the Technological Imaginary: Living and Dying in the Age of Perpetual Innovation," *Studies in Christian Ethics* 32, no. 1 (2019): 20–35; "From Anticipatory Corpse to Posthuman God," *Journal of Medicine & Philosophy* 41, no. 6 (2016): 679–95; "Of Minds and Brains and Cocreation: Psychopharmaceuticals and Modern Technological Imaginaries," *Christian Bioethics: Non-ecumenical Studies in Medical Morality* 24, no. 3 (2018): 224–45.
9 Heidegger, "The Question Concerning Technology," 296–9.
10 In CEC, the resources being unlocked, exposed, and used toward external ends are social and psychological (and perhaps economic) rather than physical. Exactly what these resources are and how they are used by various methods will be explored in Chapters 3–4.
11 Heidegger, "The Question Concerning Technology," 303.
12 Ibid., 324, italics added.
13 Ibid., 287–305.
14 Ibid., 331.
15 Ernst Kapp, *Elements of a Philosophy of Technology: On the Evolutionary History of Culture*, ed. Cary Wolfe, trans. Lauren Wolfe, Posthumanities (Minneapolis, MN: University of Minnesota Press, 2018), x.
16 Ibid.
17 Ibid.
18 Ibid., xi.
19 For example, Bernard Stiegler, *Technics and Time, 1: The Fault of Epimetheus*, trans. Richard Beardsworth and George Collins (Redwood City, CA: Stanford University Press, 1998); *Technics and Time, 2: Disorientation*, trans. Stephen Barker (Redwood City, CA: Stanford University Press, 2008); *Technics and Time, 3: Cinematic Time and the Question of Malaise*, trans. Stephen Barker (Redwood City, CA: Stanford University Press, 2010).

20. Kapp, *Elements of a Philosophy of Technology: On the Evolutionary History of Culture*, xi.
21. Ibid.
22. For an overview of the contemporary thinking of *kulturtechnik*, see Bernhard Siegert, *Cultural Techniques: Grids, Filters, Doors, and Other Articulations of the Real*, trans. Geoffrey Winthrop-Young (New York: Fordham University Press, 2015).
23. Walter J. Ong, *Orality and Literacy: The Technologizing of the Word* (New York: Routledge, 2002).
24. Notably, Ong's thesis has come under attack in recent years by sensory historians. Some argue that Ong sees too sharp a dichotomy between oral and literate cultures, a dichotomy they term the "great divide" theory. Mark Smith, for example, claims that while the print revolution certainly shifted sensory ratios such that sight became dominant, sight was highly important even in premodern societies. Additionally, sight is not as dominant as we think it is in the modern world. While I still hold Ong's work to be mostly true and important, I wonder if the emphasis on sight as the dominant sense is not completely a *modern* thing, emerging from the printing press, but a Western thing emerging from Western values and ways of thinking, out of which the printing press also was created. Mark M. Smith, *Sensing the Past: Seeing, Hearing, Smelling, Tasting, and Touching in History* (Berkeley, CA: University of California Press, 2008).
25. Ong, *Orality and Literacy: The Technologizing of the Word*, 77.
26. Verbeek, *Moralizing Technology: Understanding and Designing the Morality of Things*.
27. Ibid.
28. Jacques Ellul, *The Technological Society*, trans. John Wilkinson (New York: Vintage Books, 1964), 97.
29. Ibid., 3., italics added.
30. Ibid., 5
31. Ibid.
32. By human domains Ellul means a variety of public enterprises such as politics, economics, science, and education.
33. Ellul, *The Technological Society*, x.
34. Ibid., vi.
35. Ibid.
36. Ibid., vii.

37 Antoine Mas, quoted in ibid., 11–12.
38 Ibid., vii–viii.
39 Ibid., 21, 68–80.
40 Catherine Pickstock, *Repetition and Identity*, The Literary Agenda (Oxford: Oxford University Press, 2013), 36; for more critiques of capitalist work paradigms along these lines, see David Jones, *Epoch and Artist* (London: Faber & Faber, 2017), 143–85.; John Hughes, *The End of Work: Theological Critiques of Capitalism*, Illuminations: Theory and Religion (Malden, MA: Blackwell Publishing, 2007).
41 He writes that magic is the prototypical technique. Ellul, *The Technological Society*, 24–5.
42 Ibid., xx.
43 Ibid.
44 I am careful not to use terminology that indicates humans have complete agency over the choice, utilization, or deployment of *techne*, yet even the terminology I am using here falls short. *Techne* and human being are so intertwined that it is not quite true to say we *enlist* it for specific purposes. Rather, as we use it, *techne* helps co-determine our purposes.
45 Heidegger, "The Question Concerning Technology," 332.
46 Efficient here refers both to the quality of efficiency (achieving maximum productivity with minimum wasted effort or expense—Oxford Dictionary) and to the elevation of the efficient cause about the other three causes in Greek thought, which Heidegger identifies as characteristic of the mode of challenging-forth.
47 Iain Thomson, *Heidegger on Ontotheology* (Cambridge: Cambridge University Press, 2005), 22.
48 Pickstock, *Repetition and Identity*, 122.
49 Ashley Moyse, *Reading Karl Barth, Interrupting Moral Technique, Transforming Biomedical Ethics*, ed. Mary Jo Iozzio, Content and Context in Theological Ethics (London: Palgrave Macmillan, 2015), 105.
50 Moral strangers is originally Tristram Engelhardt's term, used to refer to those who do not share a metaphysical-moral foundation. See Engelhardt, *The Foundations of Bioethics*.
51 Moyse's words here obviously echo Jacques Ellul, Michel Foucault, and George Grant. Ashley John Moyse, *The Art of Living for a Technological Age*, ed. Ashley

John Moyse and Scott A. Kirkland, Dispatches: Turning Points in Theology and Global Crises (Minneapolis, MN: Fortress Press, 2021), 22. Italics original.

52 There is an interesting conversation in philosophy about the interplay of being and doing (or having-to-be), a conversation that grows out of a response to Kant's elevation of duty to the level of virtue. I would encourage readers to pursue these ideas further as it relates to ethicists carrying out techniques and living up to their "duties" qua ethicist in whatever systems they are beholden to. See especially Giorgio Agamben, *Opus Dei: An Archaeology of Duty* (Stanford, CA: Stanford University Press, 2013).

53 Martin Buber, *I and Thou*, trans. Walter Kaufmann (New York: Charles Scribner's Sons, 1970).

54 Generating an expression of the average is what science does best, after all; evidence-based generalizations certainly have their place but should not be confused with truth about particulars. And practical ethics is rightfully about particulars. For more on the limits of scientific reasoning about particulars, see Jeffrey P Bishop, "Intuiting the Excess: Science, Interpretation, and the Transcendence of Life," *Modern Theology* (2025).

55 Moyse, *Reading Karl Barth, Interrupting Moral Technique, Transforming Biomedical Ethics*, 106.

56 Heidegger, "The Question Concerning Technology," 331.

57 Ibid.

58 "Non-identical repetition" is a concept from Catherine Pickstock's work that I will more fully describe in the next chapter.

59 The limited data that exists with regard to the current practices of clinical ethicists suggests that larger hospitals, major and minor teaching hospitals, and hospitals connected to academic centers have more uniformity of practice and more adherence to ASBH practice standards than smaller or non-teaching hospitals. While specific methods used has not been analyzed, the existing data seems to suggest that uniformity of method is a trend that is increasing in academic bioethics and larger hospitals but is slower to arrive at smaller hospitals. Thus I do not claim that CEC has become completely standardized, because it has not (yet); however, because standardization is endorsed strongly by ASBH and academic bioethicists, I believe it is worth addressing before it becomes completely adopted into practice. See Ellen Fox et al., "Ethics Consultation in U.S. Hospitals: Opinions of Ethics Practitioners," *The American Journal of Bioethics* 22, no. 4 (2021): 19–30.

60 ASBH's recommended method is "ethics facilitation." They state: "There is general consensus in the field that "ethics facilitation" is the best model for HCEC. In characterizing this approach, we only describe its core features. We are not attempting to give a detailed model. The ethics facilitation approach is appealing in part because it can be adapted to a variety of different methods and models for HCEC (6)." Leaving aside the question of consensus in the field, it is interesting to note that according to ASBH, "ethics facilitation" includes Dubler and Liebman's Bioethics Mediation model but in some ways goes beyond it (see appendix II, 55), presumably to be flexible enough to be accomplished via various methods; yet the features of ethics facilitation are all present in the Bioethics Mediation model (see 6–8), and the section that describes these features directly cites Dubler and Liebman. It is not clear whether there are points of departure between ethics facilitation and Bioethics Mediation. I will delve deeper into this topic in Chapter 4. (See Nancy N. Dubler and Carol B. Liebman, *Bioethics Mediation: A Guide to Shaping Shared Solutions*, Rev. and expanded ed. (Nashville, TN: Vanderbilt University Press, 2011).). "Core Competencies for Healthcare Ethics Consultation," 2nd. ed. American Society for Bioethics and the Humanities (Glenview, IL: American Society for Bioethics and the Humanities, 2011), 6–8, 55.

61 Brent R. Carr, "Side Stepping the Issues: Disappointment with an Ethics Consult for a Medically High Risk Patient," *Narrative inquiry in Bioethics* 14, no. 1 (2024): 13–16.

62 Ibid., 14–15.

63 Ibid., 15.

64 Ibid.

65 Ibid.

2

What Does a Technique Do?

My loves have been automated by rituals I didn't even realize were liturgies.
—James K. A. Smith[1]

We saw in Chapter 1 that techniques are a kind of *techne*, which means that they are modes of revealing that help construct our perception of the world around us by permitting some features to emerge and hindering others. We could say that, ontologically, techniques are those processes which *co-construct with the human an ontology* of the perceived world. This construction or revealing also implies a concealing, since some aspects of reality must fade into the background as others come front and center. Yet the revealing and concealing permitted by our techniques is not only one-way; techniques end up forming us into certain kinds of people as we use them, often in ways that we do not entirely intend.

Standardized techniques, by virtue of their standardization, operate in the mode Heidegger calls challenging-forth. Many practical ethicists see no problem with standardized techniques, especially in contexts where such approaches are commonplace, like in medicine. They may even see standardization as a way of ensuring quality.[2] Thus, the goal of this chapter is to explain why challenging-forth forecloses on practical ethics. First, by exploring Catherine Pickstock's work in *Repetition and Identity*, we will see that being (both human and non-human) consists of non-identical repetitions. Then, turning back to challenging-forth, we will see how it operates with a countervailing assumption that the nature of being is *identical* repetition. As such, it allows only those features of reality which are identically repeatable to come into focus. In the realm of CEC, standardized techniques usually bring into focus a problem to be solved—a dilemma, with at least two opposing values—which, when mapped onto bioethical principles, rules, theories, etc., will correspond to an answer. Such ontological construction cannot facilitate encounter; challenging-forth enables certain other lines of inquiry but disables an encounter with being(s) (both individual beings and the interconnected system of being) as they actually are. Human beings are affected most of all, as the technique must cast them as characters in the dilemma, sometimes termed stakeholders, which limits who and what they are allowed to be. In short, standardized techniques in ethics function as *ersatz* liturgies, enabling a kind of power and control but preventing our beholding of being. I will claim that, instead, practical ethics is a search for the good, and the good is tied up with being as it is. To seek the good requires we have an ontology based on things themselves. Rather than standardized techniques, we must start with an encounter with reality and with human being(s).

Non-Identical Repetition

Humans are natural philosophizers. "To live is to construct an ontology," writes Pickstock.[3] In order to live in the world, she says, we must construct a sense of self and a somewhat stable categorization of the other things around us. Techniques are one of the ways we construct this ontology. And yet, if we start to believe that our philosophizing about things maps exactly onto the world, we will be mistaken and miss a great deal of its dynamism and surprise. We will forfeit experiences of awe and confusion, of ecstatic delight, of astonishment and reverence. We will miss something true about the world which these experiences reveal. And so, to be alive is to philosophize yet also to recognize the limits of philosophy; we must construct an ontology, but "one that must ceaselessly be revised by the vicissitudes of events and encounters, and so be rendered constantly questionable, problematic, and provisional."[4] Because the world is both classifiable and non-classifiable in its emergence, a full account of reality is one that recognizes the already-givenness of things alongside their always-arriving newness.

As we have seen, CEC techniques help us develop and work with a certain account of reality. This account of reality is, of course, one in which medical moral crises appear in a form recognizable and workable to the clinical ethicist. The operative question is: what aspects of reality are allowed to emerge as we use these techniques, and are they the aspects that are truly necessary for engaging ethical dilemmas? Do they allow us to recognize when reality exceeds our formulations and expectations, to revise our ontology "by the vicissitudes of events and encounters"? To begin to answer these questions, we must attempt a provisional ontology that can help us see beyond the limited gaze of our CEC techniques, at least for a moment, to see more clearly what it is we are engaging when we engage being(s) in moral crisis. The good—that sought by ethics—is entangled with being, with ontology.

Pickstock gives us a way into such a provisional ontology. Her first step is to interrogate the relationship between the categories of being (*ens*), essence/form (*essentia*), and thing (*res*). While Western philosophy typically prioritizes *ens* as the most basic category, within which all *res* are situated (a position called the "univocity of being"), Pickstock reverses the emphasis and focuses instead on *res* as the primary category. She focuses, in other words, on the thingness of things rather on conceptual categories about things. For this reason, she can replace ontology with "reology;" the study of things (*res*) is the study of being. Yet there is still a link missing, because we know that *res* must somehow be connected to *ens* in order to come into existence and continue in it. That link of connection is *essentia*, also called essence or form, something which is itself inseparable from the existing thing. Everything that exists participates in being through its form.

What is *essentia*, or essence, or form? In resonance with Plato's idea of the forms, Pickstock writes that every *res* has a specific nature and a mode of individuation of that nature. "This is usually described as the form of a thing, with some fluidity of the term as to whether it denotes the belonging of a thing to a general family of universal essence (this snowdrop to 'snowdrops'), or the characteristics of just this thing in particular (this green-and-white snowdrop just before me)."[5] Form links being (*ens*) together with an individual thing (*res*). An example may be illustrative. Take the human being. In Christian theology, the form of the human body (the human body being the *res* in this example) is the soul. The soul, the form of the material body, links the body to *ens*; so the human participates in being through its soul, its form, and could not exist without it. The soul is the "specific nature" of a human being, and each soul both belongs to the general family of "souls" and is completely singular as "this soul."

So things exist according to their forms. And yet, in all things except God, *res* and essence/form are divided. This means that no *res* needs to exist, and all *res* exist only by participation in *ens*. The essence/form of a thing limits its participation in being so that snowdrops, for instance, can only be snowdrops, although each has unique features. In other words,

> Nothing finitely formed in a certain specific way has to exist at all, while nothing that finitely exists has to exist just in the way that it does. . . . [This is not to say] that the cosmos might exhibit any shape whatsoever, nor that anything can turn into anything else *de potential absoluta Dei*, nor that every individually formed thing must constantly look over its shoulder, since it is in danger of losing its integrity and disintegrating into several other things (as for Duns Scotus). Rather, it is to say that everything is fluid and flexible within a certain range.[6]

Therefore, one cannot coherently separate the recognizable identity of a thing either from existence in general or from the specific location and conditions of its coming to be.

> In this sense the primacy of *res* suggests historical geography as the third metaphysical term between essence and being. *Diastasis* in space-time, or extension-duration, mediates, combines, and co-constitutes nature and being in such a way that the mark of thingness appears to be consistency and continuity despite variation. Or, in other terms, a repetition that is non-identical.[7]

While certainly difficult to get one's head around, this ontology/reology has direct implications for understanding the world. If the mark of thingness is non-identical repetition, then the category of "repetition" is the basic ontological (or as Pickstock proposes, reological) category.[8] Repetition is required for existence. Each instant we experience as "now" is already passing away. We can only identify and recognize a thing or a person when they have already been repeated from one moment to the next, i.e. held beyond the passing instant. We are always experiencing things in their emergence, in their doubling, in their slight variation from the moment before. Like rocks at the bottom of a river constantly eroding, we cannot pin down the specific characteristics of things, because they are always changing before our eyes. Techniques that rely on the pinning down of categorizable characteristics of things, without allowing them to appear new and different in each moment and context, are necessarily going to limit our engagement with being(s). Standardized CEC techniques, which insist on a dilemma-solution dyad and cast people as stakeholders within that dyad, do just that. They limit our contact with the *res*, the focus of our ethical endeavors. Our ethics, our search for the good of being, is severely constrained by this limited access to what is true about *res*, because the good is to be found in beholding things as they are.

Challenging-Forth and Identical Repetition

As we saw in Chapter 1, *techne* co-creates and enacts metaphysical assumptions that *enframe* our perception of being. Standardized techniques, which operate through challenging-forth, allow us to perceive features like reliability, direct cause and effect, and orderability in the world. While useful for certain pursuits, challenging-forth is at odds with ethical inquiry. To give further evidence, let's next explore the historical development of challenging-forth's ontology and show its departure from Pickstock's reology.

Challenging-forth is a mode unique to modern *techne*, but the type of ontological thinking that makes challenging-forth possible emerged much earlier than modern technology, in the late Middle Ages.[9] This type of ontological thinking, which set the preconditions for modern *techne* to emerge, is referred to as the "univocity of being," and it originated with Duns Scotus and William of Ockham. In direct opposition to Thomas Aquinas's earlier Medieval doctrine of the *analogia entis*, which held, like Pickstock, that humanity can only possess being by direct participation in the Divine, Scotus insisted that "being" is a concept that applies equally to God and God's creation.[10] Hence, the "univocity" of being: all things can be said to exist in the same way. No longer is God the source of being, or the source of any other transcendental, for that matter. Rather, under the univocity of being,

God, if God exists, is an entity with more attributes (or greater in degree) than humans; the difference between God and creation is a difference of quantity rather than quality.

According to Amos Funkenstein, Ockham's emphasis on the univocity of being went even further than Scotus'.[11] Ockham believed that only discrete entities exist (we can call this a radical reology), and they do not need the mediation of universals (forms, essences) for either their existence or their rationality. Ockham thus rejected the *analogia entis* completely and made the existence of God a logical non-necessity. The impact of Scotus's and Ockham's revised ontology was profound in philosophy and theology, but also in science.[12] Science in the seventeenth century abandoned the idea of similitudes in nature and embraced a system of univocal signs—essentially, mathematics.[13] No longer were things in nature understood as reflections of each other and of the Divine, such that ontology was relational and participatory. "The symbolic-allegorical perception of nature as a network of mutual references was discarded as a source for protracted equivocation," writes Funkenstein. "The image, say, of man as a microcosm that reflects and embodies the macrocosm lost much of its immediate heuristic force. Things ceased to refer to each other intrinsically, by virtue of their 'participation in' and 'imitation' of each other."[14] Now, the only system that could speak universally about things was science, the *mathesis universalis*, "an unequivocal, universal, coherent, yet artificial language to capture our 'clear and distinct' ideas and their unique combinations."[15] As a result, scientists must demand that nature be essentially, at the level of its constitutive elements, homogeneous and uniform. The same kind of matter is present in all parts of the universe, and the same laws apply to all regions and locations as long as the relevant conditions are the same. Nature is expected to display mathematical order.[16]

So, the univocity of being preceded and allowed for the rise of modern science in the sixteenth-seventeenth centuries and led to dramatic changes in the applied sciences like medicine. Much more could be said about these changes.[17] For our purposes, the important thing to note is that such incredible scientific progress[18] was made possible by a fundamental change in metaphysical thinking, from the pre-modern theological ontology of *participation* in the being of God (as Pickstock describes) to one of *univocity of being* (wherein mathematical calculations of forces are the basic building blocks of reality). The framework of the univocity of being allowed for modern science to emerge in part because it denied the transcendent and focused exclusively on matter and forces to define things. While I do not claim that a focus on matter and forces is *de facto* wrong, that matter and forces cannot define things, or that the resulting scientific and medical discoveries are undesirable, I am concerned about the effects this type of thinking has on practical ethics. Challenging-forth, synonymous with Moyse's term techno-ontology, wrongly posits *identical* repetition as the basic ontological category, meaning we are led away from the true nature of being.[19] As we saw in Chapter 1, Heidegger also sounds the alarm regarding the ontology revealed by modern *techne*, having come to see the entire history of metaphysics as a systematic neglect of being, a refusal to allow reality to emerge in itself.[20] He identifies this flattening of metaphysics to simply the actions and reactions of matter and forces (efficient causation[21]) as the project of challenging-forth. He calls us to a new attentiveness to (or we might say beholding of) being which, as Judith Wolfe puts it, "requires not so much deliberate action—since a proactive 'framing' of the world is precisely what has distorted it—as an attentive letting-be, a spiritual discipline that allows the self to become a 'clearing' on which the light of Being may fall and show forth beings as they are."[22] Perhaps we can use Heidegger's call as a starting point for inquiring about how exactly to approach being (as *res* participating in *ens*) as practical ethicists.

As we know, there are times when downplaying differences between objects is useful in medical or scientific contexts, such as when choosing between pills in a pill bottle, yet when this thinking is universalized as the only way to accurately understand things, it becomes problematic. Especially when applied to human life—the domain of practical ethics—denying difference can start to look extreme or even creepy. As Pickstock points out, dystopian novels and science fiction often play on these tropes: with a denial of non-identical repetition, life would become "a mechanical performance, reiterated from minute to minute, day to day, year to year, and any vaunted variations would perhaps be irrelevant and irregular or even illegal distractions."[23] If the differences between individual lives are ignored or downplayed in favor of their similarities, each person becomes substitutable for anyone else, and we become the typification of Ernst Junger's *The Worker*, identities reduced to our tasks.[24] We feel "docketed, tracked, and timetabled,"[25] our decisions and movements predictable and surveilled.

Indeed, this ontology is tightly connected to tasks and means of production in modern society. According to John Hughes, Karl Marx's critique of capitalism was that

> the triumph of utility is absolute and self-serving, entailing the "complete subordination of all existing relations to the relation of utility, and its unconditional elevation to the sole content of all other relations." Even "life itself appears only as a means to life." People are reduced to the status of things, living capital, the "commodity-man . . . a spiritually and physically dehumanized being" to be bought and sold.[26]

Marx observed that the elevation of utility, which is tied up with an insistence on identical repetition, "utterly abolishes the specificity of things and thus any sense of their inherent worth or value in a destabilizing that tends through an infinite regress of means and ends towards nihilism."[27] But while Marx critiques the elevation of utility for its denial of inherent worth, his materialism ultimately committed him to the same nihilism that he disavowed. Hughes notes that by attempting to secure the integrity of everything, person, and activity by making it an end in itself, Marx actually could not account for the complex relationships between things and their mutual relationship to that which exceeds them.[28] Only through an account of transcendence and participation can our ontology secure the integrity of things. Each *res* participates in a transcendent identity through its form, meaning every *res* is not just uniquely existing but is also a sign beyond itself.

David Jones, the twentieth-century artist, engraver, and poet, succeeds in uniting such an ontology with a critique of modern work and modern technology. Like Marx, Jones critiques the elevation of mere utility, or "the utile" as he calls it, but unlike Marx, Jones is able to connect his critique with an account of sign-making. Jones writes of the human as artist and sign-maker, the creature for whom all labor is inescapably sacramental and liturgical.[29] The modern world tries to deny this fact, according to Jones, bringing all life under the rule of mere utility, which is fundamentally the will to domination.

The utile is "the spirit of rationality and ruthlessness, of quantification and commodification, of sameness and indifference, of control and hoarding, opposed also to all that is ancient, particular, and differentiated, all that is free, child-like, celebratory, worshipful, cultic, holy."[30] The utile guides many of our CEC practices and procedures, which we use to rein in—to put boundaries around—the unpredictable and the chaotic, the spontaneous and free, the non-identically repeated emergence of life. Medical spaces cannot tolerate a significant amount of such unbridled emergence, and standardized, measurable, rational CEC techniques serve to limit and control it in times of conflict. According to Jones, the utile is the goal sought by "our present technocracy,"[31] alive and well in medicine, which tries to divide utility from the sacramental nature to which it has always been rightfully joined.[32]

And yet, while it can appear that the modern world is succeeding in its efforts to turn everything into "uncontaminated utility," there is a fundamental dilemma. "*If* man is the kind of creature here defined as 'man-the-artist' then none of his works can, in strict, literal fact, be wholly and exclusively ordered toward mere utility."[33] And so, Jones leaves us with the tension of two truths: humanity seeks the utile, but humanity rejects the utile. "No matter how removed we may all be [from our artistic and sacramental nature] by habit of thought and behavior and the incidence of our technocracy . . . we are still of this infantry. We were 'listed into it at birth.'"[34] We are creatures bound for art-making and sign-making, even in our rational pursuits; we are creatures in whom *Prudentia* (prudence, practicality) and *Ars* (art, gratuity) are united. Writes Jones, "Without body: without sacrament. Angels only: no sacrament. Beasts only: no sacrament. Man: sacrament at every turn and all levels of the 'profane' and 'sacred,' in the trivial and in the profound, no escape from sacrament."[35]

Without sign-making, without participation in Divine Being, without transcendence, we have the reign of the utile, the reign of the copy. But the good news, says Jones, is that our nature is not mere utility. We are each, in fact, non-identically repeated. Henri Bergson identified "mass identical repetition," associated with "mechanical reproduction," as the *enemy of things*.[36] Heidegger said something similar about modern science and mathematical reason: that it is a project of thingness which *skips over things*.[37] Challenging-forth and its techno-ontology skips over or annihilates *res* because it cannot attend to particularities. It sees identical repetitions where there are in fact non-identical ones, and as such, it cannot secure the integrity of things. The good news, then, is that there is another way.

Encounter and Being

Ethics is a search for the good of being(s).[38] In order to discover and to know what is good for any particular being, you will need to encounter them, to behold them, to engage with them as they are. The truth about being and the good for being are found together. And since beings are non-identically repeated, and historical geography is the third metaphysical term between essence and being, an encounter will require specificity. It will require embeddedness, contextuality, particularity. Concrete encounter is emphasized in the work of the New Phenomenologists—inheritors of Heidegger's and Edmund Husserl's thought—who refer to encounter as the essential ethical task.[39] Emmanuel Levinas says, "Every phenomenological experience rests upon a pre-philosophical one. . . . The encounter with the other offers us the first meaning, and in the extension of this encounter, we discover all the others. Ethics is a decisive experience."[40] But (New) phenomenologists are not the only ones to recognize the significance of encounter for ethical inquiry. German Lutheran theologian Dietrich Bonhoeffer also emphasizes concrete encounter in his *Ethics*, writing that ethical action is fundamentally

> dependent on the man who is concretely [our] neighbor in his concrete possibility. [The ethicist's] conduct is not established in advance, once and for all, that is to say, as a matter of principle, but it arises with the given situation. He has no principle at his disposal which possesses absolute validity and which he has to put into effect fanatically, overcoming all the resistance which is offered to it by reality, but he sees in the given situation what is necessary and what is "right" for him to grasp and to do.[41]

Bonhoeffer writes that no given situation should be treated like inert matter upon which we can force our ethical ideas, methods, or programs.[42] Reality, in fact, has limited receptivity for methods or programs because it does not conform to abstract universals but instead is constantly emerging.[43] "Christ teaches no abstract ethics such as must at all costs be put into practice,"[44] he writes, continuing:

> Christ did not, like a moralist, love a theory of good, but He loved the real man. He was not, like a philosopher, interested in the "universally valid," but rather in that which is of help to the real and concrete human being. What worried him was not, like Kant, whether "the maxim of an action can become a principle of general legislation," but whether my action is at this moment helping my neighbor to become a man before God. For indeed it is not written that God became an ideal, a principle, a programme, a universally valid proposition or a law, but that God became man.[45]

Thus, ethics for the Christian is "neither abstract nor casuistic, neither programmatic nor purely speculative. Concrete judgements and decisions will have to be ventured here."[46] Concrete judgements and decisions, based on concrete encounters with actual people and situations, are the work of practical ethics. The practical ethicist is "the one who sees reality as it is, and who sees into the depths of things."[47]

The point here is not to prioritize either ethics or metaphysics, but rather to insist they are *coincident* and are found in the moment of encounter with *res* itself. In an encounter with the other, our gaze as objective observer of supposedly uniform reality is interrupted. We are implicated in a reciprocal exchange in which our own ego is decentered and we become open to something new. Encounter with the other in their concreteness, in their non-identical repetition from moment to moment, allows for an existential receptivity that is a necessary stance for the practical ethicist. We participate in the circumstances of the other, not as removed expert, but as fellow human being. Rather than gaze upon reality, we behold it. Here New Phenomenology improves upon phenomenology, but still needs the addition of Pickstock's reology.

For the New Phenomenologists, encounter is different from pure phenomenological experience of things, in which pre-existing conceptions are bracketed. Phenomenology alone does not get past the Kantian divide between the mind and reality, which says we have no way of knowing whether our sense perceptions of the world correspond to the world in reality. In insisting that we bracket our metaphysics, principles, ideas, etc., to experience the thing in itself, phenomenology actually assumes the Kantian divide, the fundamental inaccessibility of the world by our minds. We will run into this problem again in Chapter 4, when we examine Richard Zaner's phenomenological method for CEC. New Phenomenology, however, is able to bring theological resources that call the whole Kantian paradigm into question and introduce the reciprocal exchange of encounter. But New Phenomenology still lacks the explicit metaphysical reorientation that would make such an exchange intelligible. When put into conversation with Pickstock's more sophisticated account of participatory metaphysics, New Phenomenology can be brought beyond its limitations and show us something important about ethical interactions—because, again, the good is intertwined with the true, and both are present in being.

Indeed, New Phenomenologists admit the limitations of phenomenology and seem to recognize the need to re-engage metaphysics. J. Aaron Simmons and Bruce Benson write that the call of the other toward encounter "always already precedes us and has both the effect of decentering us and constituting us; it is yet another example of the usual phenomenological paradigm being turned on its head."[48] Jean-Louis Chrétien says that "each new encounter shatters us and reconfigures us."[49] Unlike classical phenomenological experience, encounter is a two-way street; in encountering the other, we experience being encountered by the other. This mutuality is possible because of the mutual participation of every *res* in *ens*. While New Phenomenology has neglected to offer an account of *res* as participating in *ens* through form, Pickstock's work fills the void.

In sum, ethics is a search for the good, and it requires engagement with others in their concreteness. This concrete, contextual engagement is best described as encounter, a reciprocal exchange in which we, as ethicists, are implicated in the process of allowing situations and people to emerge. Encounter is only intelligible when supported by a robust reology that secures the integrity of all persons as participating in the being of God and existing in slight variation from moment to moment. This understanding allows us to circumvent, or transcend, the Kantian divide that would keep us all radically separate, as if inaccessible to each other entirely. Rather, we can encounter and be encountered as mutual participants in being, although never participating in exactly the same way. Being(s) and the good of being(s) coincide; metaphysics and ethics are two sides of the same coin.

An ontology of non-identical repetition helps us understand why standardized techniques, which challenge-forth, are insufficient for ethics. If being was identically repeated in all times and places, challenging-forth would be the correct mode with which to approach ethics, to encounter being and search for its good. Yet, because being is a series of non-identical repetitions, encounter with being requires being confronted with what you did not expect. Control is inimical to true encounter. Although repeatable efficacious techniques are at home in the ethos of modern medicine, because they help us see patterns and averages which can be studied systematically, ethics is a search for contextual goods and concrete decisions. It requires an openness to what we do not yet perceive, and what our procedures cannot reliably reveal.[50] Thus ethics is simply not the kind of thing that can be controlled and ensured in the same way that medicine can be (although surely medicine too exceeds our full control).

Ersatz Liturgies

Beyond the important fact that standardized techniques won't "work" for ethics because they disable an encounter with non-identically repeated reality, there is an additional problem: they function as *ersatz* liturgies. To explain what I mean by "*ersatz* liturgies" requires a bit of groundwork. First, what is a liturgy? Ritual scholar Ronald Grimes defines liturgy as "any ritual action with an ultimate frame of reference and the doing of which is understood to be of cosmic necessity."[51] Liturgy is a "technique," a rubric for action, which is aimed toward ultimate reality. Grimes does not restrict this definition to Christian liturgical rites or to just those rituals which we colloquially call liturgies. Rather, liturgy is a mode of human ritualization that contains certain key elements such as deep receptivity, reverence for the sacred, nonlinear movement, and waiting on power.[52] It involves paradoxes: in liturgy we are "acting toward inaction," and reenacting or re-presenting what can, by definition, never be repeated.⁵³ We are both speaking and awaiting permission to speak, accessing the sacred and aware that we can never fully access the sacred. Grimes identifies liturgical action, liturgical "technique," in the Christian Eucharist as well as ritual acts like Taoist alchemy, Zen meditation, and Jewish synagogue worship.⁵⁴ Importantly, liturgy takes a stance toward power not seen in other ritual modes:

> Liturgy begins with the ritual cultivation of being and is typified by a deep receptivity. . . . Liturgical power is not the force of labor, a way of achieving results, but is a mode of tapping into the way things flow or connecting with the order and reason that things manifest. Liturgy is a way of coming to rest in the heart of the cosmos. Liturgy is how a people become attuned to the way things are—the way they really are, not the way they appear to be.⁵⁵

This account of liturgy does not sound at all like the standardized techniques I am critiquing—in fact, it sounds quite the opposite. Rather than deep receptivity, which resonates with the idea of encounter explored above, standardized CEC methods approach people and situations with pre-determined forms and procedures into which cases should fit. They do not allow us to "become attuned to the way things are" because they insist on identical repetition, a false vision of reality. Clearly, standardized CEC methods are not operating in a liturgical mode.

Hence, the term "*ersatz*." Kimbell Kornu develops the idea of *ersatz* liturgies in medicine, describing *ersatz* (false, imitation) liturgies as embodied practices and stories which are fueled by moral imaginaries of the good life contrary to those of the Kingdom of God.⁵⁶ These *ersatz* liturgies function as liturgies in the sense that they form our identities, inculcate certain visions of the good life, and govern our actions. *Ersatz* liturgies, like religious liturgies, have political, formational, and affective dimensions.⁵⁷ We could say they are practices, techniques, which aim us toward *an* ultimate frame of reference, but stop short of embodying the necessary elements of liturgy as Grimes describes them.

Because standardized CEC methods form the identities of parties involved (most notably, the ethicist as ethics consultant, but also clinicians as experts, family members as stakeholders, and so on), govern political relationships within the hospital according to these roles, espouse visions of the good life, and guide future action, they function in some liturgical ways. But because they work within the mode of challenging-forth, standardized CEC methods do not contain the necessary elements of liturgy as Grimes describes. They do not allow us to see reality as it is, to encounter it fully. They do not set us up to be confronted with the unexpected, to wait on the power we cannot control or wield. Instead, standardized CEC methods attune us to a false reality of identical repetition, elevate the value of utility, and deafen us to the call of the other. Like all liturgies, standardized techniques are rubrics for worship or worshipful action; but standardized CEC methods are rubrics for the worship of false gods, especially power, control, uniformity, and progress.[58] They are situated within the biopolitical system of the hospital and exist for its benefit, which may explain why they operate with an ontology consistent with challenging-forth, the dominant mode of medicine.

For those outside of religious contexts, and those who are skeptical that liturgy is an appropriate frame through which to evaluate techniques, it may also be helpful to think of techniques as "cultural liturgies" rather than *ersatz* liturgies. James K. A. Smith, in his Cultural Liturgies trilogy, argues that liturgies are simply embodied practices, whether "sacred" or "secular," which over time shape our identities by forming our desires.[59] He famously describes how even the most secular of activities, visiting your local shopping mall, can be understood as a liturgical practice—forming your beliefs about "the good life" and about what is beautiful and worthwhile. Within the everyday cultural liturgy of shopping at the mall are found symbols, colors, images, smells, bodily movements, etc. that powerfully compel shoppers to be certain kinds of people oriented toward certain types of goods—not through convincing arguments or dogmas, but through pre-theoretical, embodied formation. Liturgical formation is a human phenomenon, not just reserved for sacred contexts. Those who do not share my understanding of Christian liturgical theology in Chapters 5–6 are thus still encouraged to evaluate the liturgical elements in their CEC techniques (i.e., their political, affective, and formational elements; their images of the good life), perhaps with Smith's "cultural liturgies" framing in mind.

In the coming chapters, we will take a deeper look at each of the common standardized CEC techniques, interrogating their alignment with challenging-forth and keeping an eye toward their liturgical elements. Building from Grimes's portrayal of liturgy and Kornu's development of *ersatz* liturgies in the hospital, we will examine the roles/identities these techniques reify, the political relationships they dictate based on those roles/identities, their implicit and explicit visions of the good life, and the types of ethical recommendations they allow. While some contain more elements of liturgical action than others, in the mode of what Heidegger calls *poiesis*, each method falls short. And even if we were to build the "ideal" CEC method, as soon as we *standardize* it, it will fall squarely under the same rubric as the others. It will become an *ersatz* liturgy, orienting us around the worship of power, control, and utility.

Notes

1 Excerpt from *You Are What You Love* by James K. A. Smith, copyright © 2016. Used by permission of Brazos Press, a division of Baker Publishing Group. Smith, *You Are What You Love: The Spiritual Power of Habit*, 45.

2 For example, see the peer commentaries in Finder and Bliton's 2018 book, including Andrea Frolic and Susan B. Rubin, "Critical Self-Reflection as Moral Practice: A Collaborative Meditation on Peer Review in Ethics Consultation," in *Peer Review, Peer Education, and Modeling in the Practice of Clinical Ethics Consultation: The Zadeh Project* (Cham: Springer Open, 2018); Anita Tarzian, "Ethics Consultation for Mrs. Hamadani - A Focus on Process," in *Peer Review, Peer Education, and Modeling in the Practice of Clinical Ethics Consultation: The Zadeh Project* (Cham: Springer Open, 2018); Lisa Rasmussen, "Standardizing the Case Narrative" in *Peer Review, Peer Education, and Modeling in the Practice of Clinical Ethics Consultation: The Zadeh Project* (Cham: Springer Open, 2018); Courtenay R. Bruce, "Not Principlism Nor Casuistry, Not Narrative Ethics nor Clinical Pragmatism" in *Peer Review, Peer Education, and Modeling in the Practice of Clinical Ethics Consultation: The Zadeh Project* (Cham: Springer Open, 2018); and Kelly Armstrong, "Telling About Engagement is Not Enough: Seeking the 'Ethics' of Ethics Consultation in Clinical Ethics Case Reports," in Finder and

Bliton, *Peer Review, Peer Education, and Modeling in the Practice of Clinical Ethics Consultation: The Zadeh Project* (Cham: Springer Open, 2018).
3   Pickstock, *Repetition and Identity*, 2.
4   Ibid.
5   Ibid., 9.
6   Ibid., 10.
7   Ibid., 11.
8   Her use of the term "reological" is interesting because brings to mind rheology, a branch of physics that studies the motion of matter. She hints at the possibility of her reology uniting metaphysics and physics, in the spirit of Aquinas, Gregory of Nyssa, Maximus the Confessor, and others who understood God as the origin and end of motion.
9   Amos Funkenstein, *Theology and the Scientific Imagination* (Princeton, NJ: Princeton University Press, 1986), 26.
10 Ibid., 26–68.
11 Ibid., 27.
12 In philosophy, the univocity of being set up the possibility for Immanuel Kant, whose importance for Western thought probably could not be overstated (see ibid., 28). In theology, the univocity of being changed the doctrines of God, creation, and providence, as well as modes of scriptural interpretation, all of which had dramatic effects (see Simon Oliver, *Creation: A Guide for the Perplexed*, Guides for the Perplexed [London: Bloomsbury, 2017], 64–132).
13 Funkenstein, *Theology and the Scientific Imagination*, 28.
14 Ibid.; for an excellent example of the macrocosm/microcosm system in a twelfth-century theologian, see Hildegard of Bingen, *Book of Divine Works with Letters and Songs* (Rochester, VT: Bear & Company, 1987).
15 Funkenstein, *Theology and the Scientific Imagination*, 28–9.
16 Ibid., 29.
17 See, for example, Steven Shapin and Simon Schaffer, *Leviathan and the Air-Pump: Hobbes, Boyle, and the Experimental Life* (Princeton, NJ: Princeton University Press, 1985).
18 By "scientific progress" I do not wish to make any claims about the trajectory of such progress. It is possible to "progress" in ways that are positive as well as negative, ambivalent, and even circular. Here I will focus instead on the progression of the relevant scientific thinking *in time*, and the implications of this modern scientific thinking on practical ethics.

19 Pickstock is equally dissatisfied with the immanentist alternative to the univocity of being (associated with Jacques Derrida, Gilles Deleuze, and phenomenologists like Husserl and his followers). She believes (and I agree) that they rely on an arbitrary bracketing of metaphysical questions, eliminating the very thing necessary for the intelligibility of every *res*—transcendence, secured by a link of the form/essence and by the process of repetition-with-a-difference. Each *res* participates in a transcendent identity through its form, meaning every *res* is a sign beyond itself, something that phenomenologists don't attend to. Pickstock's ontology's (or reology's) divergence from phenomenology will be further explored below and in Chapters 4 and 5.
20 Judith Wolfe, *Heidegger and Theology*, Philosophy and Theology Series (London: Bloomsbury T&T Clark, 2014), 138.
21 Efficient causation is just one of the four traditional Aristotelian causes, which include material causation, formal causation, final causation, and efficient causation. The efficient cause is change or movement through physical forces.
22 Wolfe, *Heidegger and Theology*, 138.
23 Pickstock, *Repetition and Identity*, 88.
24 Heidegger's views on *techne* were actually inspired by Junger's work; see Holger Zaborowski, "Technology, Truth, and Thinking: Martin Heidegger's Reading of Ernst Junger's the Worker," in *Hiedegger's Question of Being: Dasein, Truth, and History* (Washington, DC: The Catholic University of America Press, 2017).
25 Pickstock, *Repetition and Identity*, 88.
26 Hughes, *The End of Work: Theological Critiques of Capitalism*, 76.
27 Ibid., 77.
28 Ibid., 93.
29 Artist because we make things which are beautiful as well as useful; sign-maker because what we make is not just beautiful and useful but also points to a transcendent reality beyond itself. Ibid., 200.; Jones, *Epoch and Artist*, 151.
30 Hughes, *The End of Work: Theological Critiques of Capitalism*, 201.
31 Jones, *Epoch and Artist*, 181.
32 Hughes, *The End of Work: Theological Critiques of Capitalism*, 202.
33 Jones, *Epoch and Artist*, 180, italics original.
34 Ibid., 184.
35 Ibid., 167.
36 Pickstock, *Repetition and Identity*, 41.; Henri Bergson, *Time and Free Will*, trans. F. L. Pogson (New York: The MacMillan Company, 1913), 18.

37 Heidegger, "Modern Science, Metaphysics, and Mathematics," in Chap. VI In *Basic Writings*, ed. David Farrell Krell (New York: HarperCollins Publishers, 1993), 291, italics added.
38 Aristotle said, "All knowledge and moral choice grasps at good of some kind or another." Aristotle, *The Nicomachean Ethics of Aristotle*, https://www.gutenberg.org/files/8438/8438-h/8438-h.htm#chap00, Book I, Chapter II.
39 The importance of encounter is described by many great theological ethicists and philosophers, not just those listed here. It has yet to be incorporated into clinical ethics, with the possible exception of Richard Zaner, who I will explore more in Chapter 4. See J. Aaron Simmons and Bruce Benson, *The New Phenomenology* (New York: Bloomsbury Academic, 2013).
40 Emmanuel Levinas, *Is It Righteous to Be? Interviews with Emmanuel Levinas* (Stanford, CA: Stanford University Press, 2001), 160.
41 Dietrich Bonhoeffer, *Ethics*, trans. Neville Horton Smith, First Touchstone ed. (New York: Macmillan Publishing Company, 1955), 224.
42 Ibid.
43 Ibid., 71.
44 Ibid., 86.
45 Ibid.
46 Ibid., 89.
47 Ibid., 70.
48 Simmons and Benson, *The New Phenomenology*, kindle loc 1240–1248. In this section, they are describing the work of Jean-Louis Chretien.
49 Jean-Louis Chretien, "The Wounded Word: Phenomenology of Prayer," in *Phenomenology and the "Theological Turn:" the French Debate*, ed. Dominique Janicaud, et al. (New York: Fordham University Press, 2000), 156.
50 Bishop, Fanning, and Bilton, "Echo Calling Narcissus: What Exceeds the Gaze of Clinical Ethics Consultation?"
51 Ronald L. Grimes, *Beginnings in Ritual Studies*, 3rd ed. (Waterloo, Canada: Ronald L. Grimes, Ritual Studies International, 2010), 42.
52 Ibid., 42–3.
53 Ibid.
54 Ibid., 43.
55 Ibid., 42.
56 Kornu, "*Medical Ersatz Liturgies of Death*: Anatomical Dissection and Organ Donation as Biopolitical Practices."

57 Ibid.; again, note that Kornu is not contrasting *ersatz* with religious, although that is a part of the divide, but more specifically with Christian. This choice of words is mine.

58 Jeffrey P. Bishop argues something similar about spiritual assessment tools used by hospital chaplains to develop spiritual treatment/care plans. Building on Kornu's concept of ersatz liturgies, Bishop writes, "These treatment algorithms are the liturgical rubrics for spiritual therapy; they create ersatz liturgies." See Bishop, "Of Idolatries and Ersatz Liturgies: The False Gods of Spiritual Assessment."

59 Smith, *Desiring the Kingdom: Worship, Worldview, and Cultural Formation*; *Imagining the Kingdom: How Worship Works*; *Awaiting the Kingdom: Reforming Public Theology*, ed. James K. A. Smith, Cultural Liturgies (Grand Rapids, MI: Baker Academic, 2017).

3

The Four Boxes Method, Clinical Pragmatism, Bioethics Mediation, and the VA's CASES Method

Science, say Saint Augustine and Saint Thomas Aquinas, is the knowledge of things human, wisdom that of things divine. Neither their object nor their mode of being is the same. Science circulates with ease, with agility, in rivers and streams, but wisdom only wishes to drink at the source and expose itself naked, stripped of all protection, to the light alone of the perpetually new-born dawn. —Jean-Louis Chretien[1]

To fully understand why the theoretical critiques in Chapters 1 and 2 matter, we must return to the everyday doing of practical ethics. Do our commonly practiced standardized techniques exhibit the qualities of challenging-forth? What Edmund Pellegrino noted twenty years ago is still true today: "the normative power of different methodologies is an insufficiently engaged issue."[2] Here we will take a closer look at four of these methods, arranged in chronological order of their development: the Four Boxes method, Clinical Pragmatism, Bioethics Mediation, and the United States Department of Veterans Affairs' (VA's) CASES method.

These four methods vary in their goals, steps, and assumptions about the nature of ethics and ethics expertise. They vary in the ways they determine our view of reality and human being(s). But one thing they have in common is the borrowing of processes used in other fields—science, medicine, or law—to challenge-forth solutions to ethical problems. Each of these methods potentially falls prey to Ellul's critique of standardized technique in social domains: that it makes moral judgments impossible and colonizes the human body for the purposes of *techne*, purposes such as efficiency, efficacy, and repeatability. Because standardized techniques reveal to their users an ontology at odds with the fullness of being, standardized techniques turn ethics away from an encounter with being and its good, and toward the operational know-how of method deployment.

These standardized CEC methods function as *ersatz* liturgies, attuning us to a certain vision of reality. *Ersatz* liturgies narrow down the multivalent identities and interlocking relationships of their participants, revealing only the aspects of identity and relationship that serve the *ersatz* liturgy's goals. Thus, they help govern political relationships, often in ways that constrain participants into limiting roles and allow for the perpetuation of power dynamics. The types of recommendations that can emerge through the use of these techniques are constrained as a result of their revealing-concealing elements and their ritual action. They also turn backward to define the user, the ethicist, in ways that limit her ability to approximate the good, right, and true. As we examine these methods through the framework developed in Chapters 1 and 2, it will become clear that none of them are sufficient for the robust CEC that bioethicists, clinicians, and patients desire.

The Four Boxes Method

Background

The first clinical ethics technique to be articulated as a standardized methodology was the Four Topics or the Four Boxes method. It was designed by Albert Jonsen, Mark Siegler, and William Winslade and first published in 1982 as *Clinical Ethics: A Practical Approach to Ethical Decisions in Medicine*.[3] The lack of a standardized technique in clinical ethics consultation prior to the time of their writing prompted Jonsen, Siegler, and Winslade to create one, because "just as clinical cases require a method for sorting data, so too clinical ethics cases must have some method to collect, sort, and order facts and opinions raised by the ethical dimensions of the case. We have developed such a method."[4] The conviction that ethics must have a standardized technique for collecting, sorting, and ordering facts is one that already raises red flags given the argument in the preceding chapters. Collecting, sorting, and ordering facts is not sufficient for robust moral inquiry because moral dilemmas and conflicts deal in the realm of values and goods. Its emphasis on facts and order is a clue that the Four Boxes technique is aimed at challenging-forth rather than *poiesis*. Yet as we continue to examine this method's operational ontology, more concerns become evident.

The Four Boxes' vision of ethics expertise is another such concern. One underlying assumption of this technique is that clinical ethicists are clinicians alongside physicians, nurses, social workers, etc., and should operate with just as much technical precision.[5] In this schema, clinical ethics is not primarily a discipline of practical ethics, with its own expertise, in which we search for the good of concrete persons; rather, ethics is considered to fall within the domain of clinical medicine as one dimension of patient care, and therefore processes of challenging-forth should ensure quality in ethics just as they ensure quality in medicine. Therefore, Jonsen, Siegler, and Winslade write that every clinician (ethicists and others) should be able to "identify the ethical question and to reach a reasonable conclusion and recommendation for action" by using this method.[6] The technique user is interchangeable because the technique itself assures ethical action. The character, training, experience, and wisdom (or lack thereof) of the technique user is of no discernible consequence, except perhaps as indications of the individual's capacity for proper use of the technique. As noted in Chapter 1, standardized technique creates a sense of impersonality because, for the sake of consistency, the system (the hospital or the organization) relies on processes rather than on individuals. As Ellul argues, systems use standardized methods to anticipate both future difficulties and their resolutions, turning ethicists (as well as clinicians in this case) into identical and replaceable technicians of method.[7] Rather than relying on the experience, skill, and professional expertise of the ethicist, then, a system which uses a standardized technique "seeks to eliminate such variability."[8]

The Four Boxes methodology erases clinical ethics expertise in favor of technical expertise (or, perhaps, equates them), eliminating the need for clinical ethicists per se. Only in cases where a clinician is unable to resolve the issue on their own are they expected to utilize the clinical ethics consultation service, which may or may not be run by a trained clinical ethicist.[9] In either case, the Four Boxes method should be followed, as the four boxes are understood to "constitute the essential ethical structure of every clinical encounter."[10] If every clinical encounter did indeed carry an identical ethical structure, there would be no problem with the standardization of ethics technique. The problem is, of course, there is no such identically repeatable ethical structure.

Methodology

Given the background assumptions, it will come as no surprise that the methodology elaborated by Jonsen, Siegler, and Winslade straightforwardly resembles medical reasoning. The authors identify four topics or "boxes" they claim are relevant to most ethical problems in clinical practice, which can be used to "organize ethical reasoning."[11] These include (1) medical indications, (2) patient preferences, (3) quality of life, and (4) contextual features. This method structures the ethicist's attention on each of the four topics in turn, asking them to proceed through a series of questions from each in order to arrive at the best course of action. Together, the four topics

> provide a pattern for *ordering the facts* of a clinical ethical problem. Each topic can be filled with the actual facts of the clinical case that are relevant to the identification of the ethical problems. The contents of all four topics viewed together form a *comprehensive picture* of the ethical dimensions of the case. Clinical reasoning begins with the facts of the case and moves toward a presumptive diagnosis by sorting those facts into reasonable patterns of causality. *Similarly, clinical ethical reasoning starts with the facts. A statement of the ethical problem in a case follows a clear and complete collection of the facts of the case.*[12]

There is a noticeable emphasis on the facts, which when properly ordered according to the logic of the technique will provide the ethicist or clinician with an understanding of the ethical problem. This "plug and play" method should be equally effective across the entire scope of clinical ethics concerns; facts are filled into the boxes, in expectation that an understanding of the ethical dimensions of each case will emerge. This resulting understanding is said to be comprehensive, rather than limited or contingent, suggesting that users will be unaware of the way this technique structures their attention and constrains the features of the case that are allowed to emerge.

This claim to comprehensiveness and universality is apparent in the instructions for how to move through the method. Each box contains an exact set of questions which should supposedly be answered in every case. Within the first box, medical indications, users of the technique are instructed to consider "five questions that define the scope of the topic of medical indications," including diagnoses, prognoses, goals of care, probabilities of treatment success, and a medical harm/benefit analysis. Each of these elements already represents abstractions from the patient, focusing the ethicist instead on probabilities, statistics, and analyses. The second box, patient preferences, contains six questions which attempt to turn us back to the patient, covering the topics of informed consent, decision-making capacity, stated preferences, surrogates, and patient willingness to cooperate with medical treatment. Yet these framings reveal a medicalized interpretation of the patient, abstracted again from the patient-as-person. The third box contains quality of life considerations, which are supposedly captured in eight questions that are relevant to the "identification and assessment of any ethical issues."[13] These eight questions consider the prospective outcomes of treatments, the possibility of bias on the part of providers regarding the patient's quality of life, palliative care plans, and the legal permissibility of medically assisted dying and/or suicide.[14] Lastly, there are ten questions associated with contextual features. These questions relate to justice concerns in the professional setting in which consultations are occurring, settings in which various financial, business, and public interests are in play.[15]

The questions listed in each box determine and solidify the topics that are under the purview of clinical ethics as if they were straightforward and universally agreed upon. In reality, what counts as clinical ethics is constantly shifting, both in the dynamic academic literature and in practical settings. Yet the technique itself defines its subject matter and allows into CEC discourse only those ideas which are already recognized by the technique as ethical in nature. As Ellul says, "[Standardized technique] constructs the kind of world [it] needs and introduces order. . . . It clarifies, arranges, and rationalizes; it does in the domain of the abstract what the machine did in the domain of labor. It is efficient and brings efficiency to everything."[16] It is not simply the limited number of questions or boxes that indicate this method operates in challenging-forth; additional questions or categories would not assuage these concerns. Rather, any standardized methodology which imagines itself to be comprehensive will fail to capture the dynamic nature of clinical ethics and the cases for which CEC is needed.

The final step, after using the four boxes to sort facts, is to "weigh" the information sorted into the boxes so that a resolution can be reached. According to the authors, to weigh the information in the boxes against each other, and thus to weigh various bioethical principles against each other, does not imply that any principle is inherently more "weighty" than the others. Like the authors of *The Principles of Biomedical Ethics*, whose influence looms large in this method, Jonsen, Siegler, and Winslade claim that each of the four principles and therefore each of the four boxes should have equal weight. Understandably, this claim leads to confusion regarding how to proceed when principles conflict. It also leaves technique users without guidance as to the relevance of various conflicting ethical obligations represented within each box. For example, because justice includes both the individual patient as well as the wider community, both types of obligations are listed in the fourth box. Clinicians have both a fiduciary responsibility to work toward the good of their patients and a public responsibility to safeguard public health. The Four Boxes method asks users to consider various types of justice simultaneously and equally when reviewing an active case, leaving users uncertain as to how to weigh various obligations.

Perhaps anticipating these concerns, Jonsen, Siegler, and Winslade write that the resolution reached through the "weighing" of the boxes may not be clear-cut. Instead, the resolution is reached "on the whole" or "all things considered."[17] Jonsen, Siegler, and Winslade are right to consider ethics resolutions/recommendations to be contingent, inexact, and even provisional. They acknowledge that each patient is "a statistic of one," so each case is slightly different. While on these points they seem to be approaching a proper stance toward non-identically repeated persons and situations, it is unclear how their method would lead us there. Their methodology constrains ethical thinking such that only four categories of features are noticed, and these features are sorted and ordered into the structure of medical reasoning, a challenging-forth rather than a bringing-forth. With its abstracted categories, this technique does not allow for an encounter with human being(s), so it is unlikely to reveal the good. Rather, it is set up to categorize being(s) according to its own paradigm, and thus limit the kind of recommendations that can emerge.

The pragmatic weaknesses of this method are relatively transparent upon inspection. Even proponents of this method identify serious shortcomings. For example, John Schumann and David Alfandre admit,

> The straightforward listing of the topics tends to lead to oversimplification of the ethical points of a case. In addition, it is often challenging to operationalize the four topics into a cogent approach to clinical ethical decision making. Once the points and questions are arranged into their respective topics, it may be difficult to know where to begin to move forward in the decision-making process. [18]

Oversimplification of complex ethics cases is a troubling feature of this method. Even more surprising, though, is its failure to offer a "cogent approach to clinical ethical decision making." The Four Boxes method structures a procedural approach to information-gathering that resembles medical decision-making and does not *necessarily* assist in the development of an ethical recommendation. This lack of guidance in how to move toward normative decisions leaves users of this method wondering how to proceed at the end. Schumann and Alfandre suggest, "Often, the best starting point is to identify one to three options that can be presented to the patient/surrogate to prompt a discussion of the preferences of the patient and the patient's family."[19] But this seems to be moving in circles, simply bringing the consultant back to box two.

While pragmatic critiques like these are important to note, it is the method's operational ontology that should be most heavily critiqued. Again, as Ellul writes, pragmatic critiques place us squarely back in the logic of standardized *techne*, where we compare rival techniques and judge them in terms of "what is useful rather than what is good. Purposes drop out of sight and efficiency becomes the central concern."[20] Practical shortcomings could conceivably be worked out, for instance, by combining this method with others that provide more guidance on ethical deliberation, yet the underlying beliefs motivating this method (i.e., that ethics is about ordering facts) would continue to make an ethical encounter impossible.

Regardless of pragmatic solutions, the Four Boxes technique would still function as an *ersatz* liturgy. Its liturgical character places people into their respective roles—physician, nurse, patient, surrogate—and governs the political relationships between them. The technique user, having taken all twenty-nine questions into account, is vested with the authority to recommend a course of action which is ethically authoritative. A vision of the good life is assumed and demonstrated: a good life is one of balance between the four principles, and thus the four boxes, where methodical information gathering and reasonable, rational deliberation sufficiently guide action. This *ersatz* liturgy, performed in specific steps in a specific order, ensures the medical system can continue to operate without calling its own gaze or methodology into question. The medical gaze is extended into the domain of ethics.

A conflation of ethical knowledge and processes with medical knowledge and processes results in a misunderstanding of what is possible and desirable in a CEC technique. As we have seen, techniques are modes of revealing that shape our gaze and make us into certain kinds of people. Ideally, a CEC technique is a provisional world-constructing practice that reveals the good to and for humans on the brink of decision. Yet when CEC techniques are made in the image of medical techniques—in the mode of challenging-forth rather than *poiesis*—they are world-constructing practices focused on reliability, repetition, efficiency, and usability. They determine for the user what counts as ethics for the purpose of problem-solving. They frame the ethical question or dilemma more like an illness which can be resolved with proper diagnosis and treatment than an opportunity for robust and messy moral dialogue. When standardized, the Four Boxes method will tend to pull us counterproductively away from ethical reflection on the good of concrete persons and toward the values of modern *techne*: primarily efficiency, efficacy, and repeatability. The method will preserve our gaze as objective observer of uniform reality, rather than allowing for a "reciprocal exchange" [21] in which our ego is decentered. The Four Boxes technique makes impossible the existential receptivity that is a necessary stance for the practical ethicist.

Clinical Pragmatism

Background

The Clinical Pragmatism method, when standardized, will also tend to pull us counterproductively away from ethical reflection on the good of concrete persons and toward the values of modern *techne*. This method, created by Franklin Miller, Joseph Fins, and Matthew Bacchetta, is a derivative of Deweyan pragmatism[22] and is built upon two pillars: "the pragmatic method of ethical inquiry," which readers will recognize from the Prelude, and "the democratic model of clinical practice."[23] Its version of pragmatic ethical theory is closely tied to utilitarianism: it aims to promote benefit, minimize harm, and engage in an analysis of proportionality.[24] In order to reach these aims, it takes as normative a democratic process of moral deliberation and consensus building. The authors combine these commitments to form a method consisting of four steps: (1) assessment, (2) moral diagnosis, (3) goal setting, decision-making, and implementation, and (4) evaluation of the results.

At the heart of Clinical Pragmatism is the belief that clinical ethics ought not to be principle or theory-driven, but rather responsive to actual problems as they emerge in healthcare. For reasons described in the Prelude, I sympathize with the move to more pragmatic approaches in clinical ethics, especially against the backdrop of the philosophical movements of the 1980s and 1990s. Clinical Pragmatism's methodology was first articulated in 1996, in direct response to these movements. Miller, Fins, and Bacchetta write, "Susan Wolf recently argued that bioethics is undergoing a shift in paradigm from 'principlism,' which has shaped the mainstream of the field from its inception in the late 1960s, to pragmatism. . . . We endeavor . . . to contribute to the articulation of the pragmatic paradigm for bioethics . . . "[25] An important function of bioethics is to help determine how best to meet the needs of concrete persons in clinical settings. Theory alone will not do.

Clinical ethics is thus described by Miller, Fins, and Bacchetta as a discipline that brings processes of moral inquiry (rather than static moral norms) to bear on healthcare practice, allowing for each to be revised in light of the other.[26] "The process model of moral problem solving is inherently dynamic;

it concerns interactions between clinicians and patients (or surrogates) in a relational process with a trajectory extending into the future."[27] The process is likened to the image of a corkscrew:

> The linear thrust of the corkscrew represents the teleological movement of inquiry from a problematic situation to a satisfactory resolution, following the steps.... Participants engage in continuing cycles of forming and testing hypotheses aimed at figuring out what is going on, deciding what to do, intervening experimentally, and evaluating the results. This in turn may lead to reappraisal of the problem and a new cycle of diagnosis, planning, and intervention.[28]

This self-adjusting approach seems very similar to the practical ethics I described in the Prelude and which I take to be normative. Yet, upon further inspection, there are crucial differences.

For one, Clinical Pragmatism insists on a problem-solution dyad. As seen in the quote above, this method needs each CEC to contain a "problematic situation" and a "satisfactory resolution," the latter being reached by following the method's steps. "Clinical ethics is concerned," say the authors, "with analyzing and resolving moral problems . . ."[29] This formulation is set up to reveal moral dilemmas as problems which can be solved satisfactorily if only the method is used correctly. It constrains what is noticeable to ethicists, revealing the information that is useful for resolution and concealing information that may hinder it. Because it has a teleological end point, the image of the corkscrew suggests that ethical deliberation always has deliverables and a point of termination. This thinking is not native to practical ethics, which has for its image a circular feedback loop rather than a corkscrew. Rather, this dyadic thinking is part of the logic of modern *techne*.

Further, the philosophical foundations of Clinical Pragmatism—based in John Dewey's pragmatic philosophy—contain the assumption that ethics, like science, is a domain that can be empirically verified. The terminology of the quote above makes this easily apparent, with words like experiment, hypothesis, and intervention. Miller, Fins, and Bacchetta write, "Since moral beliefs should be considered as fallible, they have the logical status of hypotheses, not certain laws or self-evident truths. Dewey saw profound implications for the reconstruction of ethics and social philosophy in applying the logic of experimental inquiry to moral problems of social life."[30] While the approach described sounds dynamic and flexible, the standardized process for clinical ethics that results from the assumption that ethics is empirically verifiable is much more inflexible than it appears at first. The Clinical Pragmatism technique adopts a medico-scientific method of problem solving (assess, diagnose, implement, evaluate) for CEC, which disables free and full ethical engagement with emergent realities in favor of efficacy, repeatability, and ensuring forward motion toward a solution. It thus makes impossible the receptivity and disruption that are necessary for ethical encounters.

Dewey's desire to integrate science and ethics through his pragmatic method of experimental inquiry grows from an understandable dissatisfaction with the dualisms of modern thinking:

> I became more and more troubled by the intellectual scandal that seemed to me involved in the current (and traditional) dualism in logical standpoint and method between something called "science" on the one hand and something called "morals" on the other. I have long felt that the *construction of a logic*, that is a *method of effective inquiry*, which would apply without abrupt breach of continuity to the fields designated by both of these words, is at once our needed theoretical solvent and the supply of our greatest practical want.[31]

It seems that Dewey's search for a "theory of everything" leads him not so much toward theory as toward modern *techne*. Dewey turns to the power of method, the logic of technique, to unify the disparate ontologies at work in modern science and ethics. As we have seen, this strategy can indeed "supply our greatest practical want," but not without some serious compromises to moral thinking.

Finally, pragmatism's insistence that "whatever works" should be normative reflects a technocratic approach to ethics that I believe is misguided. Attention to concrete realities is an essential aspect of practical ethics, and practical ethics is "pragmatic" in the sense that real-world possibilities limit or constrain ethical deliberation. But practical ethics is also constantly looking beyond the merely pragmatic, imagining new moral possibilities. It grounds normativity, right and wrong, in goods and values rather than what will "work" in a given situation. The thing that "works" in an unjust system will be unjust. Pure pragmatism risks overlooking, perpetuating, and even commending existing power imbalances, social inequities, and bias. For Dewey and thus for the creators of Clinical Pragmatism, " . . . 'method' consists of logical patterns of inquiry that promote successful problem solving," and *not* a "process consisting of rules for discovering 'Truth,' for understanding reality, or for determining right from wrong."[32] In fact, "There was no moral system at work in Dewey's ethical thought."[33] Instead, Dewey's moral philosophy consists of only (1) the validation of ethical judgments through the logic of empirical technique, and (2) moral principles as hypothetical tools in the deployment of empirical-moral technique.[34]

Beyond its failure to ground normativity, pragmatism in clinical ethics risks a type of hubris that disables ethical inquiry. An engineer may operate with an epistemological pragmatism—knowing that exhaustive knowledge of tools and materials is impossible yet remaining unconcerned because exhaustive knowledge is not required to get the job done. This version of pragmatism seems to be assumed by many clinical ethicists as well, because decisions must be made with limited knowledge and time. But there are crucial differences between the engineer's work and the clinical ethicist's work. Practical ethics is a discipline that must be aware of what exceeds it in order to be done well; awareness and appreciation for what we cannot reliably and empirically verify is a necessary element, because goods, like being, surpass our understanding. Practical ethicists know that their work is inhibited by lack of access to the fullness of being, bringing a stance of humility and receptivity, a deliberate refusal to grasp for control. Since ethics is a search for the good of being(s) that are always just beyond our grasp, it is only possible when we are aware of (and concerned by) the limits of our grasp. To imagine we have everything we need for a workable solution based on pragmatic fact, especially when that workable solution is molded from an identically repeatable technique, is to forfeit a necessary stance of humility.

While there are some helpful aspects of the Clinical Pragmatism technique—particularly its nuanced understanding of the relationship of theory to practice, its dissatisfaction with dualisms, its appeal to the internal goods and norms of medicine, and its attempt to elevate the agency of patients—its approach ultimately disables robust ethical inquiry. It claims to give attention to the particularity of cases, but Clinical Pragmatism is ultimately unable to attend to particularity while it challenges-forth solutions to ethical problems. Like the other methods in this chapter, Clinical Pragmatism's *poiesis*-like elements are taken up into the work of challenging-forth.

Methodology

Like the Four Boxes technique, "Clinical pragmatism understands moral problem solving as proceeding according to the same method of inquiry as clinical problem solving."[35] It makes sense, then, for this clinical ethics technique to follow the same "schematic outline" as that of medicine. First is the moral assessment, in which the ethically relevant factors are identified and evaluated. The assessment must include:

> relevant medical facts; the life situation of the patient; the patient's capacity to make health care decisions; the beliefs, values, preferences, and needs of the patient; the impact of the care of the patient on family members and others intimately concerned with the patient; institutional arrangements that may be obstructing shared decision making; the perspectives of involved clinicians; and relevant moral, legal, and institutional norms.[36]

These factors, while more numerous than what is required for the Four Boxes method, are still quite limiting. Nevertheless, these factors count as the necessary and sufficient source material for the next step, the moral diagnosis. The nature of a moral diagnosis is not explicitly stated, but it seems to be something that emerges naturally for the ethicist after assessing all the relevant information from step one.

The third step is to determine appropriate goals of care with the patient and/or family. Goal setting should integrate medical and ethical knowledge, be collaborative among all stakeholders, and take place in a "climate of open, patient, and empathetic communication to facilitate adequate understanding of the patient's condition, and to prepare the patient or surrogate for meaningful participation in the medical decision-making process."[37] Possible courses of action are articulated and discussed among the stakeholders, and the decision-making process proceeds according to both medical and moral judgments, operating in tandem. A decision is made about what to do, and this decision is understood as an "experimental intervention" aimed at resolution of the moral problem. Framed this way, ethics concerns are the moral equivalent of a physical pathology, on which clinicians intervene. Finally, the plan is implemented and the results are monitored and evaluated.

The types of knowledge and ways of knowing permitted by this method are slightly more expansive than the Four Boxes method. Here users are encouraged to attend to more perspectives than their own and to facilitate meaningful participation among stakeholders. Yet, the facts and values elicited are still plugged into a medico-scientific process, with the effect of creating a workable problem-solution dyad. The method's creators admit this when they say, "By integrating ethical and clinical thinking, the method of clinical pragmatism is serviceable to clinicians and ethicists."[38] The information relevant to problem solving is put into workable form, and the information that could compromise the telos of the technique, a satisfying solution, is excluded. And all of this is in service to serviceability.

As an *ersatz* liturgy, Clinical Pragmatism delimits roles and relationships. In addition to a problem-solution dyad, this technique also reifies a "clinician-patient (or surrogate) dyad."[39] In recent years, scholars have brought attention to this oft-assumed dyad, calling into question its accuracy and usefulness.[40] What about, for instance, cases where capacitated patients refuse to advocate on their own behalf or make decisions about their care but defer to family members?[41] What about patients who are mentally ill or disabled and have fluctuating capacity for decision-making, requiring periodic assistance from family or friends? In cases where a surrogate decision-maker is present, should surrogates be considered a complete stand-in for the patient, or is decision-making a three-way conversation between clinician, patient, and surrogate?[42] What about when a surrogate is suspected of being abusive toward the patient? Or, if nursing staff express different perspectives from the physician, should they be allowed to enter into the decision-making? These questions merely scratch the surface, yet it is clear that the complexity of medical decision-making, especially in moral crises, exceeds the traditional clinician-patient (or surrogate) dyad. Relationships, even those that are truly dyads such as marriages, are always entangled with other relationships outside the dyad. The relational dynamics of family systems are complex and become even more so when interfacing with the (complex and hierarchical) relational dynamics of the medical system. To isolate relationships in ways that are intelligible to this CEC method (clinician-patient, patient-surrogate, physician-stakeholder, etc.) constrains each person's voice and their mode of participation in the case, for good or ill.

Clinical Pragmatism's liturgical action also inculcates a certain vision of the good life, one in which all stakeholders participate in a democratic process of decision-making. This good life is communal, reasonable, and verbally articulate. More importantly, it is pragmatic: the good is what works for everyone, not what is ideal or theoretical. There are certainly benefits to all of these features, yet it is important to acknowledge what is concealed or forbidden by this image of the good life. The reliance on democratic models of decision-making, where each rational agent advocates for their own interests, often veils existing power dynamics rather than challenging them. Democratic approaches privilege the articulate, the logical, and the verifiable, and marginalize somatic or emotional ways of knowing, as well as tradition-based and cultural ways of knowing.[43] We often engage in democratic processes of decision-making out of a desire to hear and give space to diverging points of view, yet just as equality does not ensure equity, democratic processes do not ensure everyone around the table is given proper levels of agency or authority.

Dewey observes that "life is a moving affair in which old moral truth ceases to apply."[44] This is in some ways true because life consists of non-identical repetitions, and moral truth must be reinterpreted or reapplied in new situations. The authors of Clinical Pragmatism are correct to note, "In the face of problematic situations, it cannot be presumed in advance that a given moral rule or principle should guide conduct. . . . The nature of the situation needs to be surveyed; all the relevant moral considerations bearing on it should be brought to light and evaluated."[45] Yet Dewey and the creators of this method are mistaken about the way forward; just as our ethical theories and principles fail to capture the "moving affair" of life, so too does standardized *techne* fail to get at reality as it is. Our techniques, like our theories, will block our access to the "relevant moral considerations" if they are taken to be static and infallible rather than provisional, revisable, and flexible. In short, we must engage practical ethics dilemmas with *poiesis*.

Bioethics Mediation

Background

Bioethics Mediation is arguably the most well-known and widely practiced CEC method today.[46] It could also be considered the most professionally self-serving method for clinical ethics consultants. Developed as a cohesive methodology by Nancy Dubler and Carol Liebman in 2004 and updated in 2011, Bioethics Mediation has proven heavily influential for the ASBH's professional recommendations for clinical ethics consultants. While the *Core Competencies* report stops short of telling ethicists to use Bioethics Mediation, the second and latest edition advocates for all of the elements of Dubler and Liebman's methodology.[47] In fact, Dubler was a member of the Task Force that created the second edition of the *Core Competencies*. The report states,

> Bioethics Mediation is a well-tested conflict resolution technique. It combines the clinical substance and perspective of clinical ethics consultation with the tools of the mediation process, using the techniques of mediation and dispute resolution to promote a principled resolution, compatible with the principles of bioethics and the legal rights of patients and families.[48]

The Task Force characterizes Bioethics Mediation as combining CEC with the *techne*—tools and techniques—of mediation to achieve CEC's goals. The problem, I will show, is that the adoption and standardization of mediation techniques for CEC do not achieve CEC's goals (which are actually goods, not goals); in fact, the adoption and standardization of these techniques disable and distorts moral inquiry. Bioethics Mediation avoids some of the pitfalls of the methods that borrow scientific processes to challenge-forth solutions to problems. Yet, it falls into other traps and remains in disjunction with the purposes of ethical inquiry.

First introduced by Nancy Dubler and Leonard Marcus in 1994, Bioethics Mediation was officially developed as a systematic and teachable method in 2004 by Dubler and legal mediator Liebman.[49] One major concern Dubler and Liebman raise as an impetus for their book is the lack of prescriptive guidance to help train new clinical ethics consultants. Approaches were not standardized enough at the time for new ethicists to learn them efficiently. By 2004, Dubler had been testing out Bioethics Mediation with her clinical ethics colleagues for many years; they had become convinced that "by far the most effective and efficient way" to gain the interpersonal and process skills required for CEC "is to study the body of knowledge, skills, and techniques represented by the field of [legal] mediation." Once again, ethicists look to the *techne* of other disciplines to remedy the inefficiencies of non-standardized ethical inquiry. Of the five reasons given, four are logistical: mediation is a technique that can be taught, mediators are available to train ethicists, mediation can address growing administrative and insurance-related conflicts, and mediation can reduce litigation.[50] While ethics terminology such as goods, values, truth, virtues, and harm are glaringly absent, Bioethics Mediation is identified as effective, efficient, teachable, and cost-saving—all ideas that reflect the values of modern *techne*.

Besides logistical ease, why mediation? Why did Dubler and her colleagues leave behind the skills and processes internal to practical ethics and find what they believed to be better skills and processes in the field of mediation? One answer is that the consults they were engaging on the ground repeatedly presented as conflicts which could be mediated. Therefore, the skills and processes of mediation appeared to be exactly what was needed. "A decade of observation had arrived at a theory:" they write, "bioethics disputes are essentially conflicts, and the underlying issues of patient and family rights can best be clarified and addressed by approaching the turbulence and discord with the skills of dispute mediators."[51] Mediation doesn't just work, but even enhances CEC because "it acknowledges the primacy of rights and the complexity of interests in medical care decision making. It recognizes the differentials in power and authority that pervade the medical setting. Most important, it has established skills and a body of knowledge that can be brought to bear on . . . disputes."[52] In other words, the theory behind

Bioethics Mediation is that bioethics is essentially composed of conflicts between autonomous rights holders. Like the other CEC techniques, Bioethics Mediation thus sets up the conditions under which its own technique will be effective. Frame CEC as a conflict between rights holders, and the technique of conflict mediation will resolve it.

Yet another answer to the question "why mediation?" is that clinical ethics has lacked standardized processes and metrics by which it can be evaluated. Dubler and Liebman are legitimately concerned that the integrity of CEC has been left largely up to the goodwill and sensitivity of individual consultants. Without quality measures, whether or not a patient ends up with a "good" CEC outcome can seem like a matter of luck. They write that in the age of patient safety and quality improvement, no medical function should be exempt from rigorous review.[53] Yet, as we know, the field of bioethics still lacks consensus regarding the most crucial questions that would undergird any effort to measure quality, i.e., what is ethics quality? What is ethics expertise? How should ethicists interact with their institutions? Where does authority lie? To whom is the ethicist beholden? And the list goes on. The Preface to *Bioethics Mediation*'s second edition states,

> A major part of the problem [with ensuring quality] was lack of consensus in the field in regard to how bioethics professionals should be trained and evaluated. There had been some discussions over the years directed at the education and status of clinical ethics professionals, including the [ASBH's *Core Competencies* report] ... [but] none of the proposals for training and evaluation have yet reached a level of acceptance in the bioethics community that would permit progress on this front.[54]

Of course, things have progressed on this front since 2011 (namely, the HEC-C credentialing program launched in 2018, which relies heavily on ASBH's Core Competencies and ASBH's ethics facilitation approach). But even now we cannot claim a consensus in bioethics regarding the appropriate training and evaluation, [55] and even the basic questions of our field remain contested. In the absence of disciplinary or professional consensus, as we have seen, many have turned to procedural benchmarks. Dubler and Liebman did the same, writing that "If the field was not going to police itself" then institutions were going to need measurements by which to evaluate CEC, the easiest of which are procedural.[56]

Before detailing the methodology of Bioethics Mediation, Dubler and Liebman discuss the differences between their CEC method and legal mediation. There are seventeen differences listed and explained, such as "The bioethics mediator is generally employed by the hospital," "The playing field is usually uneven for patients and their families," "The parties usually do not sign agreements to mediate," and "The person with the greatest stake in the dispute, the patient, is often not at the table."[57] As the long list of differences unfolds, one wonders in what sense Bioethics Mediation can be called mediation.

Lawyer and mediator Haavi Morreim, leader of the Center for Conflict Resolution in Healthcare LLC, argues that Bioethics Mediation fails to meet mediation's three primary principles of ethics and process.[58] These principles include confidentiality, neutrality, and self-determination. Each is necessary in order to build clients' trust, which is crucial for the success of the mediation process.[59] Bioethics Mediation, however,

> curtails *confidentiality* by requiring that any information regarding a patient must be passed along to providers, regardless of whether the patient consents. [Bioethics Mediation] abridges *self-determination, inter alia,* by expecting the mediator at least sometimes to enforce an agreement even if one or more parties no longer endorse it. Finally, *neutrality* is infringed as BEM [Bioethics Mediation] requires mediators unilaterally to limit parties' options. Parties will only be permitted to make agreements that lie within the range of "clearly accepted ethical principles, legal stipulations, and moral rules defined by ethical discourse, legislatures, and courts . . . " That is, the mediator will not allow parties to choose any option outside those boundaries.[60]

Because of these breaches, Bioethics Mediation risks (1) missing the underlying issues because parties often will not share without a promise of confidentiality, (2) a *"bullied acquiescence*—the reluctant 'yes' that might eventually come when someone simply doesn't want to discuss a matter further"[61] and (3) the ethicist getting dragged into an existing fight. All three are severe logistical barriers to CEC, but more importantly, they are serious ethical violations.

Moreover, Morreim shows that Bioethics Mediation as currently articulated actually *cannot* be true mediation. Morreim offers a distinction between two types of ethics consults which are conflated by the Bioethics Mediation method: those which require moral guidance and those which need conflict resolution.[62] While some consults need both types, moral guidance and conflict resolution are distinct in purpose, process, and outcome. Her clarity on the difference between moral guidance, which includes genuine ethical inquiry into the good of/for persons, and conflict resolution, which serves to help parties stop arguing, sheds light on some of the reasons Bioethics Mediation is problematic. Bioethics Mediation combines the two—using (stripped down) mediation techniques from conflict resolution to yield moral guidance—something Morreim recognizes as a category error. "In mediation, someone who is not part of a dispute helps parties find their own resolution. The mediator does not take sides or steer parties toward a preferred outcome . . ."[63] whereas clinical ethicists should steer parties toward certain decisions and away from others.[64]

Morreim shows that the Bioethics Mediation method is ultimately ineffective at best and manipulative at worst. However, her corrective is not to leave mediation to legal departments. Instead, she writes that ethicists and others should employ ("course-corrected") mediation in CEC *and more widely throughout* healthcare organizations, but "where mediation is used, it needs to be the real thing."[65] Interestingly, in arguing that ethicists course-correct their mediation practice, Morreim admits that even effectively implemented mediation is not a sufficient approach to clinical ethics as traditionally defined. Mediation techniques won't work for the traditional purposes of CEC (ethical inquiry, moral guidance) qua practical ethics. Thus, Morreim would have us carve up clinical ethics expertise into two categories: moral guidance or ethical inquiry, the skills and processes for which she does not address, and the additional practical service of conflict resolution, a legal expertise with legal skills and processes. In fact, this additional service should and does retain its own internal goods and core principles of practice and ethics (confidentiality, neutrality, and self-determination) even though those goods sometimes run counter to the ones that allow for ethical inquiry. And yet these two are supposed to co-exist in the practice of CEC.[66]

Morreim correctly describes the failures of Bioethics Mediation to live up to the ideals of mediation, which harms involved parties and undermines conflict resolution. She is also correct about the mismatch between the purposes and techniques of mediation and those of practical ethics. In fact, Morreim shows that if an ethicist is going to practice CEC well, she will be unable to meet the professional and ethical requirements to which mediators are held (neutrality, confidentiality, etc.). However, she leaves unanswered the question of how to approach the "moral guidance" type of CEC, which is outside the mediation purview. Therefore, practical ethicists still need to answer the question of technique.

Methodology

Bioethics Mediation contains eight stages, but Dubler and Liebman are careful to say that the division of steps is an artificial process, and that events in real cases never proceed in a predictable and orderly manner.[67] Mediations are not linear; participants may circle back to earlier stages, and some steps may even be eliminated. The authors aim to provide "suggestions . . . and enough theory to guide the variations."[68] So far, this sounds like a sufficiently flexible method for CEC. Yet in a predictable response to this flexibility, the authors emphasize that understanding the goals of each stage (the expected outcomes) and correctly performing the micro-techniques necessary to accomplish those goals are paramount. Thus, the closer one looks, the less flexible the technique appears.

The eight stages include: (1) assessment and preparation, (2) beginning the mediation, (3) introducing the patient, (4) presenting and refining the medical facts, (5) gathering information, (6) problem solving, (7) resolution, and (8) follow-up. This technique's *ersatz* liturgical action reliably guides users from the chaos of conflict to an agreeable solution; it narrows and solidifies identities and governs political relationships between parties. Bioethics Mediation ensures forward motion from (conflictual) problem to (amenable) resolution, even if stages must be repeated or reiterated along the way, like Clinical Pragmatism's corkscrew. This technique constructs a world in which ethics concerns or quandaries are conflictual problems between interested parties, and the technique user (the ethicist-mediator) is a neutral facilitator who can coax agreement out into the open. Bioethics mediators play multiple roles throughout the process in order to realize this identity, explain Dubler and Liebman: convener, amplifier, coach, guide, process manager, information gatherer, referee, seeker of common interests, facilitator, reality tester, empathizer, norm enforcer, staff educator, and impartial party.[69] While some aspects of these roles seem appropriate for practical ethics, some are not, and the lack of native ethics language is troubling. Ethics language is especially hard to introduce in this method because ethics consults are framed as conflicts between rights holders (which they often are, yet they always far exceed such simplification). By virtue of this framing, the professional identity of the ethics consultant becomes subsumed under the overarching identity of mediator and its sub-roles on the way to resolution. These factors create an environment in which participants' identities and relationships too are constrained to fit the permitted narrative, as they are in any standardized technique.

As the details of each stage unfold, the method reveals itself to be a confusing blend of ethics-related tasks and legal mediation strategy. In stage one, ethicists complete such preliminary tasks as assessing the situation, evaluating the nature of the dispute, gathering information about the medical and decision history of the case, and meeting with involved parties. They also prepare for the mediation, which includes identifying the legal decision-maker, choosing who to invite to the table, and arranging a location. While this stage is flexible to context within a certain range, it starts to *enframe* the ethicist-mediator's perception of the consult so that they see the elements necessary for mediation (opposing parties and their interests, a neutral setting in which to elucidate them, etc.). In identifying the legal decision-maker, for example, the technique user narrows the confusion of multiple authorities and valid perspectives, not to mention interconnected webs of influence and shared decision-making, down to one person, making decision-making more straightforward. Bioethics Mediation will certainly tolerate some disagreement, but it searches for common interests in service of eventual unanimity, aimed ultimately at resolving interpersonal conflict and ending with a solution that makes all parties happy.

This technique's use of persuasion toward consensus can be well-meaning and productive, especially when shared interests do exist, but in intractable dilemmas it can be harmful and controlling. Ethicist Ashley John Moyse presents a challenge to Bioethics Mediation's prioritization of certain modes of speech and reasoning: rather than transforming conflict into a genuine agreement, Moyse says the technique coats dissenting voices in a thin veneer of consensus.[70] Power is not equalized; it is wielded—often in ways that are hidden behind ritualization and decorum. Efficient methodologies aimed at moral conflict resolution turn us away from the call of those before us, toward the authority of systems which demand a consensus in all but the most extreme circumstances.[71]

Stages two through seven occur within the mediation itself. First, mediators carefully set the scene with introductions, provide an opening statement (detailing the mediator's role, the process, goals, disclosure of previously received information, ground rules, limits of confidentiality, and what will happen at the end), and give an opportunity for questions. Of course, this stage has the benefit of being easy to teach and to memorize, but it also constrains the kind of communication that can take place. Unlike some other aspects of the method, this part is heavily standardized because setting the scene is crucial for reaching eventual resolution. In other words, allowing the technique to *enframe* our attention in a certain way ensures that we will end up in the place the technique allows (agreement, or in rare cases when agreement cannot be reached, escalation to another department). Leaving aside Haavi Morreim's critiques of this stage qua mediation, we should note that ethics language and intention are glaringly absent here. Of course, finding shared interests and correcting miscommunication for the sake of resolution is an ethical activity. Yet more robust dialogue about goods and values may be difficult in the atmosphere created by opening statements emphasizing processes, goals, disclosure, and confidentiality. More importantly, it seems rare that such an atmosphere facilitates a genuine encounter with being(s) and a mutual, reciprocal search for being(s)' good.

In stage three, the family is invited to introduce the patient, who is often troublingly absent from the mediation. Dubler and Liebman instruct technique users to complete this stage before engaging the medical team in hopes of alleviating some of the power imbalances between medical providers and family members. While the medical team and the ethicist-mediator benefit from a huge power differential in this setting, letting the family introduce the patient first helps to level the playing field—or at least, that is the intention. When this stage allows for a holistic understanding of the patient-as-person to emerge, it may permit the patient and/or family's vision of a good life to surface. It may encourage a more equitable distribution of authority and credibility between the family and care team. It may even approximate an encounter between persons. However, as a step in a standardized process that challenges-forth a solution, these goods will likely be swallowed up by the machinery of the method. The standardization of the method already forecloses on the possibility of these goods altering the trajectory of the technique, leaving them without much relevance besides their factual merit.

In stage four, the medical team is asked to describe the patient's medical history, the current medical facts, and the prognosis. This initial description "provides a common base on which to build future discussions."[72] Indeed, a common base is erected at each stage of this technique, as it slowly reveals a reality that all parties can agree on and excludes aspects of reality that cannot be reconciled. Facts are given prime real estate. Dubler and Liebman admit the medical facts are never purely objective and that they are often difficult to establish, especially in a room with diverse perspectives on the situation. Yet "the bioethics mediator brings a unique epistemological filter" and "a successful mediator must process the information provided and help the parties evaluate their own positions realistically *against a normative notion of reality*."[73] It is unclear exactly what the ethicist-mediator's unique epistemological filter is, except perhaps the one permitted by their CEC technique. Techniques are indeed epistemological filters—or in Heidegger's words, modes of revealing. As we use them, a certain world is constructed for us. "Successfully" using the epistemological filter of this *techne* seems to mean putting in order the relevant facts and positions and compelling participants to measure themselves against the normative notion of reality endorsed by the *techne* itself. Dubler and Liebman do not elaborate on the content of this normative notion of reality, but we can assume it contains the boundaries of legality and any bioethical norms the consultant believes are relevant and justified. It also likely reinforces the view that conflicts are occurring between autonomous rights holders but can be solved with rational discourse; thus, the world is one that makes sense and can be reasonably ordered when all parties get on the same page. Those who find themselves outside this normative notion of reality, who believe, for example, that the bioethical norm does not apply or the conflict cannot be reasonably resolved, are asked to "measure themselves," perhaps to find themselves wanting and correct their views to meet the standard. While stage three was concerned with elevating the agency and perspectives of the family (successfully or not), stage four's enforcement of a vague normative notion of reality could easily undermine such efforts.

The fifth stage involves gathering further information from each party present at the mediation. The ethicist-mediator invites each party to speak without interruption while listening for the interests, feelings, and perceptions behind their words. This way of opening up the conversation seems like it will promote understanding and dialogue. However, through the use of micro-techniques of conflict resolution, the ethicist-mediator must shape the conversation according to the goal of the method, which is agreement. Thus, "Using the techniques and tools [of mediation], the mediator helps the parties create a mutually acceptable definition of the problem and of the issues and interests that should be discussed. Only when the parties agree on what the problem is can they begin to work toward a creative solution."[74] The directive to find a "mutually acceptable definition of the problem" can constrain ethical discourse such that important details are excluded if they are not universally acknowledged. Defining the "problem" (and again, here the technique's *revealing* action is aimed at "problems") in a way everyone can agree on can *conceal* the perspectives of those with less power or influence, or simply those with views unshared by others.

Ethicist-mediators are also encouraged to use the conflict resolution microtechnique of acknowledging feelings. When participants get overly emotional about the case, ethicist-mediators are encouraged to "help the parties deal with their emotions" so that the mediation can continue. Simple acknowledgement may suffice, i.e. "Dr. Post, it sounds like you are very concerned about patient Benson and it is hard to find his family so angry and mistrustful."[75] When participants remain angry or upset, "the mediator may have to direct the participants' attention away from emotive behavior if it is not moving them toward their goals."[76] But whose goals are thwarted by emotion in the mediation? It seems more likely that strong emotion thwarts the process of the technique, and the corresponding goals of the ethicist-mediator, rather than the goals of the upset participant. Bioethics Mediation asks its users to redirect or downplay the emotions of those involved so that it can move forward unthwarted. One of the characteristics of a successful outcome in Bioethics Mediation is that it "allays the anxiety of the patient or family, to the extent possible, and directs attention to the medical choices being faced."[77] Allaying the patient and family's anxiety can be a feature of good CEC, or it can reflect a CEC that is emotionally manipulative. If allaying emotional distress is a step on the way to the overarching goal of a rational decision that parties can agree on—rather than an end in itself—it is likely emotionally manipulative.

Similar concerns extend into stages six and seven, where problem solving and resolution development are the primary objectives. Mediators are to help the patient and family "understand the medical facts, assimilate the possible consequences, measure the range of outcomes against shared values, and evaluate and choose options in response to medical questions."[78] Certain micro-techniques, including managing the discussion, developing options, shaping solutions, and helping parties make choices, assist in these goals. At the resolution stage, the technique allows three options: (1) parties reach agreement on all issues, (2) parties decide they will not reach agreement and the case is escalated, or (3) parties plan for another session to allow more time for agreement to form. The mediator's role is different in each situation, but the goal remains an agreeable solution. In the final stage, the ethicist-mediator follows up on the case, oversees the implementation of the resolution, and reviews relevant hospital policies.

Along the way, ethicist-mediators should be employing various micro-techniques taken from classical mediation. Some have already been mentioned, but there are quite a few more, such as summarizing, reframing, questioning, dealing with power imbalances, generating movement (via asking problem-solving questions that keep the discussion moving toward a solution), stroking (both recognizing feelings and recognizing participants' efforts in the mediation), normalizing, and focusing on the future. There are multiple ways to view the use of these techniques in CEC; on one hand, since Dubler and Liebman offer them as options rather than mandates, they may be flexible enough to aid the ethicist in the creation of a legitimately open and fruitful moral space. On the other hand, these techniques risk being taken up into the challenging-forth that Bioethics Mediation encourages, where even well-meaning interactions serve the heavy-handed petition for a resolution. It is important to remember that each CEC method contains some laudable qualities, yet their standardization reveals to their users the efficient and efficacious rather than the good. In the case of Bioethics Mediation, it takes a lot of discernment and nuance to be able to recognize both the good qualities of the technique and the dangers of its deployment across all contexts.

A Note on ASBH's Ethics Facilitation Standards

ASBH does not currently mandate any particular standardized method for CEC, but it does recommend an approach to CEC that it calls "ethics facilitation," which so closely resembles Bioethics Mediation that it is worth discussing here. Ethics facilitation claims to be compatible with a variety of different standardized methods—presumably, any of the five discussed— because it is a general professional standard rather than a method itself. It comprises a group of skills and processes guided by a normative definition of CEC and its attendant goals.[79] While many of these elements are outside the scope of my argument, it is worth acknowledging that ethics facilitation rests on many of the faulty background assumptions that give rise to standardized techniques, and it mistakenly advocates for the use of standardized techniques at the local level. The *Core Competencies* states,

> The use of standards, or standardization, has a negative connotation to some people. However, for any healthcare service, a certain degree of standardization is essential to ensuring quality. Process standards are especially important for services like HCEC, where quality cannot be determined merely by assessing the final outcome or product.[80]

As was made clear in the Prelude, this perspective reflects the contemporary misconception that ethics can be divorced from metaphysics and united instead to procedural correctness; as we've eroded the *what* from clinical ethics we've simultaneously strengthened the *how*. But standardized processes and procedures are not neutral vehicles to good normative conclusions. In fact, they have normative pull away from robust moral inquiry aimed at the right and the true.

While I do not wish to oppose all forms of standardization in clinical ethics so that there is no recognizable practice at all (more on this in Part II), I have challenged the assumption that ethical quality can be ensured through standardized *procedures*. We have seen that in fact, standardized procedures warp ethical inquiry; as Ellul says, they make moral judgments impossible. They reveal a world that is predictable and orderable, enabling a certain kind of power and control, but disabling free, full, robust moral deliberation. Yet ASBH advocates for this kind of standardization, writing further, "To competently perform an HCEC, a thorough and systematic process is essential. A sound consultation process should include explicit stages. . . . The HCEC service should have clearly identified methods for these steps."[81] The problem, as we continue to see, is that systematic processes ultimately disable ethical inquiry by challenging-forth rather than bringing-forth, and by approaching being(s) as identically repeatable rather than always redoubling anew.

Additionally, while ASBH claims that ethics facilitation is flexible enough to be accomplished via any standardized method, its procedures and outcomes align so closely with Bioethics Mediation that the two can be difficult to distinguish. In fact, nothing ASBH recommends is at odds with the Bioethics Mediation method, but if any other method were to be used, it would need to be modified. Ethics facilitation and Bioethics Mediation attempt to realize the same two-fold ideal: to stay within the bounds of scholarly literature and legal and bioethical standards,[82] and to follow a process that respects all parties and increases the likelihood of consensus. To reach consensus, ASBH recommends the Bioethics Mediation protocol for formal meetings where conflict exists.[83] The only discernible difference between ethics facilitation and Bioethics Mediation is that the former is less specific about standardized methodological requirements and offers additional recommendations for consults that don't fit the mold of conflict resolution (such as curbside consults and policy review).

Ethics facilitation, as a set of professional practice guidelines, is not subject to the same critiques as standardized methods. Yet because ethics facilitation advocates for the use of a standardized method and aligns with one problematic method in particular, ethicists have cause for concern. Whatever its merits, ethics facilitation as currently articulated is insufficient for practical ethics because it demands the use of a standardized technique for moral inquiry, revealing an underlying misunderstanding of the nature of this work. Standardized techniques cannot attend to particularities and cannot facilitate an encounter with being(s). Moreover, they constrain our view such that we unwittingly wield power and control rather than participate in reciprocal moral encounters. Thus, while it may go a long way toward creating a shared vision for the profession of clinical ethics, insofar as it utilizes standardized techniques, it will create ethics technicians rather than ethicists. It will cause us to increasingly fail to attend to the reality of being(s) in moral crisis. Ethics facilitation can be an acceptable approach to CEC only if it resists the use of standardized techniques and gets clearer about what exactly practical ethics is and does. We must re-situate CEC in the field of practical ethics united with metaphysics, rather than in the fields of medicine, science, communications, or law. CEC is rightfully a search for the good of being(s), requiring techniques in the mode of *poiesis*, with the capacity to reveal to us the subject of moral inquiry: non-identically repeated human being(s).

The VA's CASES Method

Background

Finally, we have another standardized process created in an attempt to secure quality in ethics. The VA's CASES method was designed by the National Center for Ethics in Health Care to "standardize the process of ethics consultation throughout the VA system."[84] It is part of the IntegratedEthics Program, launched in 2007 to "disseminate a systems-focused model to promote and improve ethical practices in health care—and *a new way of thinking about ethics*."[85] CASES is an acronym for the five steps of this consultation method:

(1) clarify the consultation request, (2) assemble the relevant information, (3) synthesize the information, (4) explain the synthesis, and (5) support the consultation process. Consultants are required to follow all steps in the method when engaged in active clinical cases and encouraged to follow it for consults not directly related to active cases as well, even when it seems that some steps are not required or relevant to the case. "We intend these steps to be used similarly to the way clinicians use a standard format for taking a patient's history, performing a physical exam, or writing up a clinical note," reads the primer. Therefore, "... each step should be considered systematically as part of every ethics consultation."[86]

Because the authors intend for it to be used systematically and across the VA system, this method is probably the most currently standardized and standardizable of the methods. And in the eyes of many, the implementation of a system-wide standardized process for CEC makes the VA a "recognized leader in quality and organizational change."[87] The VA is lauded by the academic community and news media alike for its success in providing exceptionally high-quality medical care when compared to other hospital systems; according to the developers of CASES, the implementation of a standardized approach to CEC is an outgrowth of the same drive for quality.[88] As explored in the Prelude, one of the underlying motivations for standardization in CEC is the unexamined belief that there is a *right* way to do it—a normative "how" of CEC—such that *quality* coincides with *uniformity*. The assumption that a standardized technique will yield a quality result is seen clearly in the VA's IntegratedEthics program and its CASES method.[89] But what exactly counts as quality ethics is left largely unexamined; it is briefly described as practices that are consistent with "widely accepted ethical standards," something that arguably does not exist.[90] Making things even more murky, while the goal of IntegratedEthics is to "*improve ethics quality* in health care," the stated goal of ethics itself is "to *improve health care* by facilitating the resolution of ethical concerns."[91] So the IntegratedEthics program and its CASES method improve this undefined thing called ethics quality, which is good insofar as it improves health care quality. More specifically, according to the articles the VA cites, ethics improves *efficient* and *cost-effective* health care but does not have any effect on the medical outcomes of patients. In fact, the cited studies claim that no difference in medical outcomes was noted between control groups and those in which CEC was performed, but CEC decreased futile or costly end-of-life care (costs which redound largely to the VA). In sum, the evidence they provide in favor of CEC is not that it improves moral decision-making, or even that it improves health outcomes, but that it decreases inefficient, costly, or futile health care in ICU settings.[92] "Health care quality," then, which CEC is set up to improve, seems like health care that serves the interests of the VA and perhaps incidentally serves the interests of some patients.

So it seems that in the IntegratedEthics program, ethics is in the service of efficient delivery of health care, an instrumentalization that not only bypasses the question of what counts as quality ethics (only tying it up with "quality health care," itself tied up with financial interests), but even explicitly views ethics as a cog in the wheel of the medical system. Good moral decision-making often does make health care cheaper and more efficient, but to equate the two is painting with too broad a brush at best. At worst, equating ethics with cheaper and more efficient health care delivery instrumentalizes ethics for the financial benefit of medical institutions. In other words, CASES represents an ethics procedure that challenges-forth cost savings.

There is more evidence to suggest this method instrumentalizes clinical ethics for the smooth functioning of the medical system. Another reason given for pursuing quality in ethics is that unresolved ethics concerns can lead to burnout and high turnover among staff.[93] When ethics concerns are addressed, staff productivity and efficiency are improved. And finally, the VA claims that "failure to maintain an effective ethics program can seriously jeopardize an organization's reputation, its bottom line, and even its survival."[94] While high-quality CEC may benefit the organization in a number of ways, if organizational benefit and protection are the only reasons given for maintaining an ethics consultation service, it is reasonable to conclude that CEC is operating in the mode of challenging-forth. Ethics ought not to be seen primarily as a means by which to protect the organizational system. The instrumentalization of ethics procedures toward the ends associated with challenging-forth should raise a red flag for practical ethicists, as should the lack of normative vocabulary. Words such as "morals" and "goods" are conspicuously absent.

Methodology

In order to understand more specifically which aspects of reality are brought into view by this method and which are hidden by it, it will be helpful to explore the details of the CASES technique. It should be kept in mind, however, that whatever the features of an ethics technique, as soon as it becomes standardized, it is already functioning in the mode of challenging-forth. The further details of the technique's revealing-concealing action only add to its insufficiencies.

The first step in the CASES method is to clarify the consultation request, which involves characterizing the type of consultation request, obtaining preliminary information from the requester, establishing realistic expectations, and formulating the ethics question.[95] A primary goal in this step, captured by the instruction to "characterize the type of consultation request," is to determine whether the request is actually an ethics concern or is best suited for another department. While this seems like a natural first step for any approach to CEC, and may be somewhat unavoidable due to the siloed nature of medical systems, it has the effect of severing ethics from the contextual elements arising simultaneously in which ethics becomes relevant, elements which are by definition intertwined with ethics. In other words, the first step in this technique is to constrain reality such that ethics concerns or questions are conceptually and practically distinct from the context in which they arise. The instructions state, for example, "Often requesters who are seeking legal advice want assistance resolving an ethical concern (uncertainty or conflict about values) as well. When a question involves both legal and ethical concerns, the legal aspect should be referred to legal counsel and the ethical concerns addressed by the ethics consultation service."[96] Far from benign, this dividing up of interrelated concerns to different departments constrains and *enframes* the ethicist's perception of the situation in ways that disable a genuine encounter with the full features of a consult from the very beginning.

Once the ethicist has determined the consult to be directly and solely related to ethics, they are required to gather information from the requester in six specific areas: the requester's contact information and title, urgency of request, brief description of the case and ethical concern as the requester understands them, requester's role vis-à-vis the case, steps already taken to resolve the ethical concern, and the type of assistance desired.[97] Notice what types and sources of information are left aside by this information gathering, and what types and sources are deemed important and relevant. The perspective of the patient is initially set aside, for example, while the perspective of the requester sets the frame for the construction of the ethics consult.[98] Notice how the requester (likely in this formulation to be a concerned member of the medical team) is in charge of the narrative, and is reified in the role of concerned professional. The ethicist's role begins to take shape as professional supporter of the medical team, revealing the technique's assumptions about ethics expertise. What is more, these six brief informational categories *enframe* the ethicist's attention such that they are equipped to formulate chaos, uncertainty, and conflict into a concise ethics question that fits one of the following two structures:

Given _____ (uncertainty or conflict about values) _____, what decisions or actions are ethically justifiable?

Given _____ (uncertainty or conflict about values) _____, is it ethically justifiable to _____?

The possibility of more than one ethics question in a single consult is acknowledged, as well as the possibility that the ethics question(s) may evolve or require modification throughout the consult. "Nevertheless, formulating the central ethics question at the outset is essential, as it helps to focus subsequent steps."[99] Indeed, this formulation functions as a device to limit our attention and exclude what is considered extraneous so that the method can go on and ultimately arrive at its concluding point unthwarted.[100] The content of moral dilemmas becomes fodder for the operation of the technique itself, rather than the other way around. In other words, the technique does not conform to the specific realities of the case, assisting moral deliberation, as much as moral confusion is made to conform to the technique. A short case study may illuminate the problems caused by the need to "formulate the ethics question" before engaging in an ethics consult. This narrative was relayed to me by a fellow clinical ethicist:

> Our ethics committee receives a call from the children's hospital to help with Jessica, a 17-year-old frequent patient who has an eating disorder. Jessica

is on the autism spectrum, and she refuses to take in liquids by mouth, demanding to have a PICC line deliver her fluids. However, a PICC line is only a short-term solution, and therefore the medical team is questioning if it is appropriate to transition to a port. Additionally, Jessica's parents want her to have a feeding tube. However, Jessica is verbally and clearly opposed to a feeding tube. She refuses to see psychiatry and refuses to call her condition a mental illness. She is adamant there is something biologically wrong with her that prevents her from tolerating fluids by mouth. Jessica also frequently picks at her PICC line, causing infections. Jessica is in the hospital every month or so—she refuses to drink by mouth, and gets so dehydrated that she needs to be admitted. The doctors are vocal about their frustration that there is "no solution" to her condition while also feeling frustrated that she refuses to see psychiatry for what they believe is a fully psychological problem.

When the ethics committee is first consulted, two team members spend time discussing how to categorize the ethics question. On the one hand, ethics consultants are not supposed to tell clinicians how to practice medicine—so it did not seem right to weigh in on the safety or efficacy of a port or G-Tube. Should the consult be refused? On the other hand, there seemed to be questions of adolescent informed consent and refusal to see psychiatry, which are ethical in nature. The team spends about 10 minutes saying "what's the ethics question?" over and over, and things like "This doesn't seem to be our problem, it seems like the medical teams don't want to do the work and are putting it on us."[101]

By the time the ethics committee successfully sorts through the multiplicity of details to find those directly under the purview of ethics and formulates a single ethics question to focus their deliberation, it is likely that the question will no longer capture the complexity of the case. The crucial concerns related to the placement of a G-Tube, for example, will be extricated from the backdrop of Jessica's affect, her parents' frustration, her autism, her history with medical interventions, and other realities that don't fit into the formula for an ethics question. The process of extraction that results in a single ethics question not only distracts ethicists from the full picture, using valuable committee time just to discern "the ethics question," it also constrains the ethicists' focus once they begin the consult such that they are only able to comment on the narrow selection of topics on which bioethics has traditionally been considered authoritative, i.e., informed consent and informed refusal, best interests, and so on. Additionally, such constraint serves to reify the identities of the persons gathered, as all liturgies do—here, doctors as medical technicians and ethicists as bioethical technicians in a supporting role.

Next, ethicists are encouraged to gather data from four sources: the patient, the health record, staff, and the patient's family members and friends, "in a thorough and systematic manner."[102] This involves carefully verifying the accuracy of this data, since "the quality of an ethics consultation depends on the accuracy of the information collected,"[103] and being sure to distinguish facts from value judgements.[104] There is little acknowledgment of the multivalent nature of narratives, especially those heard from many points of view. This step constructs a reality in which facts are cleanly distinguishable from values; and even though the preceding step was careful to identify values as the purview of ethics, this step hints at accurate facts being the source material for ethical judgments and values being distractions for the ethicist. I worry this step unintentionally privileges systematically verifiable forms of information—those types which are the sources for medical knowledge—rather than the socially embedded, multiplicitous, and embodied forms of knowledge that are the most crucial for practical ethics. In the operation of this step of the technique, a particular form of reality emerges, narrowing the ethicist's attention toward careful verification of source data and mistrust of perspectival narratives.

Step three in the CASES approach is to synthesize the information gathered in an effort to address the ethics question as formulated in step two. Ethicists should determine at this stage whether a formal ethics meeting among stakeholders is required. Since formal meetings are "inefficient" and "logistically difficult and time consuming" to arrange, they are not encouraged for every consultation.[105] The authors of CASES also point out that many patients and families are uncomfortable speaking in a group of medical professionals in a formal ethics meeting and may feel intimidated. Rather than viewing this as an imbalance of power worthy of being addressed and critiqued, the authors of CASES see it as an inconvenient hindrance to the efficacy of the formal meeting, and thus recommend assembling as much information as possible without a formal meeting, only holding one if necessary. If a formal meeting is determined to be necessary, ethicists are encouraged to follow the meeting framework laid out in Bioethics Mediation.[106]

Another element of the "synthesize" step is to engage in ethical analysis. It is here that flexibility, nuance, and expertise are allowed to guide the ethicist:

> Ethics consultants should not rely exclusively on a single approach to ethical analysis; rather, they should draw on a broad repertoire of approaches and incorporate elements of multiple approaches as appropriate when analyzing a single case. Familiarity with a range of theoretical perspectives provides the consultant with a variety of different lenses to "combine and shift" in order to unpack tough ethics questions.[107]

The theoretical approaches suggested shortly after, however, are rather narrow: principlism, casuistry, and "other approaches" including feminist ethics, rules-based approaches, and narrative ethics. While the encouragement to engage multiple theoretical approaches when conducting ethical analysis goes some way toward encouraging complexity and nuance, as one step within this standardized technique, the allowance is still too small. Embedding ethical analysis within a system of challenging-forth severely constrains moral possibilities. When the "problem" is portrayed in a prescribed format—a single-sentence ethics question—and information carefully sorted through and verified for factual accuracy and direct relevance to recognized ethics topics, ethical analysis has already strayed too far from the concrete situation. An ethical encounter with being at this stage will be very unlikely.

Steps four and five include communicating the synthesis and recommendation(s) to key participants of the consult, documenting the consult with precision in the health record, following up with the case, and evaluating the consultation process. In their evaluation of the consult, ethicists are encouraged to "compare actual processes followed to established standards," i.e., the steps and requirements of the CASES method, and to self-correct any deviations from the logic and procedures of the technique. In the final stage, ethicists are to elicit feedback from participants and are told to adjust processes as necessary, which sounds like it is in line with *poiesis*. Yet, feedback should be gathered via a (standardized) assessment tool, and VA employees must "follow policy requirements and procedural standards when seeking feedback."¹⁰⁸ Even the part of the technique that encourages feedback and adjustment is operating in challenging-forth.

CASES is a practical, step-by-step technique that standardizes consultation across the entire VA healthcare system in an attempt to secure ethics quality. Like the other CEC methods, it makes the complex and often overwhelming responsibility of ethics consultation seem manageable, repeatable, teachable, and sustainable. Yet, this method overtly applies challenging-forth to the process of CEC by borrowing and modifying processes from science and medicine for the purpose of practical ethics. This has the effect of allowing only certain aspects of reality to emerge as relevant to ethics and structuring a consult into a single-sentence ethics question that can be answered by careful documentation and theorizing. It reifies roles and identities which are necessary for the efficient carrying out of the technique (i.e., physician as medical technician, ethicist as bioethical technician). By aligning their CEC method with the way clinicians use efficient techniques, standardized *techne*, to bring about repeatable results, the developers of the CASES method prioritize efficacy, repeatability, and quality control over encounter and disruption. The types of recommendations that will be permitted by this technique are ones in line with such values.

Like a liturgy, this method contains several steps which must be carried out in a specific order with a specific purpose. It is a rubric for action, it forms identities with political and formational dimensions, and it encourages a certain orientation toward the good. But it is *ersatz*, in the sense that it trains us in ways that run counter to genuine worship; it is an embodied practice that aims us away from receptivity to the unknown and toward the organization and molding of reality into workable forms. In short, this *ersatz* liturgy puts the ethicist in charge of wielding their institutional power to overcome the ethical dilemma and support the medical team.

The procedures or techniques we use for CEC have implications for the meaning assigned to "ethics" and to the ways dilemmas appear to us. By turning CEC into a technical enterprise rather than a participatory work of conscience, a certain frame is created such that the impetus for "ethics" is an ethical "problem." The emergence of an ethical "problem" or "question" sets in motion the institutional mechanism by which health care operationalizes a response, the mechanism being CEC and the response being a solution/recommendation. The ethical "problem" recognizable to the institutional machinations of procedural CEC often does not even resemble what Mark Bliton and Stuart Finder call the "bristling thicket of emotions and face-to-face interactions that frequently provide clues" to the actual values and goods that are the object of ethical inquiry. Bliton and Finder write,

> The characteristic assumption at the organizational level is that the function, the job, of ethics consultation is to make these sorts of problems recognizable as "typical," and then to use standardized expectations, policies, norms, and so on to explain how and why to respond. With that reliance on standardized expectations, policies, and procedures for conducting clinical ethics consultation, the focus shifts from talking about the moral reasons and actions that prompted those expectations, policies, procedures, and so on, in the first place to the effective fulfillment or completion of the designated procedures, so that "ethics" because a set of procedures performed in an accountable way.[109]

The four methods explored in this chapter are examples of this kind of thinking. Each responds to the organizational pressure for procedure by borrowing processes from the domains of science, medicine, or law to ensure predictable results in CEC. They attempt to secure quality in secularized medical contexts where normativity is contested by standardizing the approach and the technique.

In the next chapter, we will examine an approach to CEC that eschews standardization and attempts to facilitate an encounter: Richard Zaner's Phenomenological Method. Zaner's approach is praiseworthy for its rejection of scientific, medical, and legal techniques in CEC. His method is squarely situated within philosophical ethics. Because it is not proceduralist, it is better able to resist power dynamics and overly simplistic characterizations of stakeholders' interests. It tries to attune us to lived reality, to center the patient through a phenomenological account of illness, and to make ethics responsive to context. Yet, as I will show, even this more nuanced method fails in its metaphysical assumptions about being(s). Even Zaner's method falls short of enabling a robust and normative ethical encounter.

Notes

1. Used with permission of Fordham University Press, from Jean-Louis Chretien, *Under the Gaze of the Bible* (New York: Fordham University Press, 2014). Permission conveyed through Copyright Clearance Center, Inc. Jean-Louis Chretien, *Under the Gaze of the Bible*, ed. John D. Caputo, trans. John Marson Dunaway, Perspectives in Continental Philosophy (New York: Fordham University Press, 2015), 41.
2. Pellegrino, "Bioethics at Century's Turn: Can Normative Ethics Be Retrieved?" 662.
3. The information in this chapter is taken from the latest edition, the 9th edition: Albert R. Jonsen, Mark Siegler, and William J. Winslade, *Clinical Ethics: A Practical Approach to Ethical Decisions in Clinical Medicine*, 9th ed. (New York: McGraw Hill, 2022).
4. "Introduction," ibid.
5. Ibid.
6. Ibid. There is an ongoing debate in the clinical ethics literature over whether "ethics expertise" exists, and if so, what it is. While I do not wish to dive deeply into this debate, it is worth noting that the authors of the Four Boxes method (as well as Clinical Pragmatism) seem to adopt the stance that clinical ethics has no expertise on its own outside of medicine. Clinical ethics is rather, for them, a part of responsible medical practice. Under this view, clinical ethicists would not be necessary if physicians and other clinicians were adequately formed in the ethical dimensions of their work. I acknowledge this stance as a legitimate answer to the question of ethics expertise; however, the adoption of medical processes for the ethical dimension of medical care is still inadequate for the task. It reveals a fundamental misunderstanding about the nature of moral inquiry and the nature of being, even if clinical ethics were to be understood as essentially linked to the practice of medicine rather than a practice with its own internal goods.
7. By identical, I mean identical for the purposes of the system or identical in the ways relevant to their function within the system. Ellul, *The Technological Society*, 11–12.
8. Ibid., 67.
9. "Introduction," Jonsen, Siegler, and Winslade, *Clinical Ethics: A Practical Approach to Ethical Decisions in Clinical Medicine*.

10 Ibid.
11 Ibid.
12 Ibid., italics added.
13 "TOPIC THREE: Quality of Life," ibid.
14 It is troubling that questions about the legality of physician assisted suicide (PAS) and suicide are raised in every clinical ethics consultation. Even in cases where these two topics are relevant, the placement of these two questions at the end of the "quality of life" box might suggest that unfavorable quality of life assessments should result in the active consideration of PAS. In any case, the last questions in any list are often the most memorable and top of mind. I would argue that PAS and suicide should not be top of mind for ethicists in the category of quality of life considerations.
15 Question 6 is a curious additions to this box. It asks, "Are there religious factors that might influence clinical decisions?" One would expect religious factors to surface in Box Two, Patient Preferences, rather than here, unless this question is referring to the religious commitments of healthcare institutions such as Catholic hospitals. Even so, the inclusion of this question in a box that is focused on justice amidst conflicts of interest seems to suggest that religious factors hinder ethical decision-making in unjust ways, or work against the development of just decisions. These subtle suggestions may be intended or unintended, noticed or not, yet they influence the thinking process of the technique user.
16 Ellul, *The Technological Society*, 5
17 Jonsen, Siegler, and Winslade, *Clinical Ethics: A Practical Approach to Ethical Decisions in Clinical Medicine.*
18 John H. Schumann and David Alfandre, "Clinical Ethical Decision Making: The Four Topics Approach," *Seminars in Medical Practice* 11 (2008): 42.
19 Ibid.
20 Ellul, *The Technological Society*, vii.
21 Catherine Pickstock, *After Writing: On the Liturgical Consummation of Philosophy*, ed. Gareth Jones and Lewis Ayres, Challenges in Contemporary Theology (Oxford: Blackwell Publishers, 1998), 176–7.
22 For more on Deweyan pragmatism, see John Dewey, *The Political Writings* (Indianapolis, IN: Hackett Publishing Company Inc., 1993); *The Philosophy of John Dewey*, ed. John J. McDermott (Chicago, IL: University of Chicago Press, 1981).

23 Franklin G. Miller, Joseph J. Fins, and Matthew D. Bacchetta, "Clinical Pragmatism: John Dewey and Clinical Ethics," *Journal of Contemporary Health Law & Policy* 13, no. 1 (1996): 29.
24 J. J. Fins, F. G. Miller, and M. D. Bacchetta, "Clinical Pragmatism: Bridging Theory and Practice," *Kennedy Institute of Ethics Journal* 8, no. 1 (1998): 37–42.
25 Miller, Fins, and Bacchetta, "Clinical Pragmatism: John Dewey and Clinical Ethics," 27.
26 Ibid., 28.
27 Ibid., 47.
28 Ibid., 34.
29 Ibid., 28.
30 Ibid.
31 John Dewey, *From Absolutism to Experimentalism* (1929–30), in *2 The Philosophy of John Dewey: The Structure of Experience* 1–13 (John J. McDermott ed. 1973), reprinted in *5 John Dewey: The Later Works*, 1925–1953 (Jo Ann Boydston ed, 1981), 156, quoted in ibid., 32, italics added.
32 Ibid., 35.
33 Ibid.
34 Ibid., 36.
35 Ibid., 49.
36 Ibid., 48.
37 Ibid.
38 Ibid., 49.
39 Ibid., 29.
40 For example, M Kuczewski, "Reconceiving the Family: The Process of Consent in Medical Decision Making," *Hastings Center Report* 26, no. 2 (1996): 30–7; Rebecca Dresser and John Robertson, "Quality of Life and Non-Treatment Decisions for Incompetent Patients," *Law, Medicine & Healthcare* 17, no. 3 (1989).; Emmanuel and Emmanuel, "Proxy Decision-Making for Incompetent Patients," *JAMA* 267, no. 15 (1992): 234–44.
41 Anita Ho, "Relational Autonomy or Undue Pressure? Family's Role in Medical Decision-Making," *Scandanavian Journal of Caring Sciences* 22, no. 1 (2008): 128–35.
42 Linda Post, Jeffrey Blustein, and Nancy Dubler, "The Doctor-Proxy Relationship: An Untapped Resource," *Journal of Law, Medicine & Ethics* 27, no. 1 (1999): 5–12.
43 Miller, Fins, and Bacchetta claim that Dewey's pragmatism does not privilege logic over emotion, because Dewey rejected the Kantian cognition/emotion

dichotomy. Emotion, for Dewey, offers moral insight which can be used as empirical data points in pragmatic inquiry just like logic. To me this indicates that Clinical Pragmatism puts emotion into the category of data, to be used and ordered just like scientific knowledge, which implies an instrumentalizing that still privileges logical ways of knowing. See Miller, Fins, and Bacchetta, "Clinical Pragmatism: John Dewey and Clinical Ethics," 38.

44 John Dewey, *Human Nature and Conduct* (New York: Cosimo Classics, 2007), quoted in Miller, Fins, and Bacchetta, "Clinical Pragmatism: John Dewey and Clinical Ethics," 39.

45 "Clinical Pragmatism: John Dewey and Clinical Ethics," 41.

46 See Haavi Morreim, "Mediating in Healthcare's Clinical Setting: Time for a Course Correction," *Ohio State Journal on Dispute Resolution* 35, no. 1 (2019): 90.

47 There seems to have been some debate among members of the ASBH Core Competencies Task Force as to whether ASBH's ideal model, which they term "ethics facilitation," differs from Bioethics Mediation. They clarify in Appendix II that Bioethics Mediation is necessary but not sufficient for their vision of CEC: "The term "mediation" was not mentioned in the first edition. Some would state that bioethics mediation contains sufficient expert knowledge to justify its own category, but the Task Force decided that mediation knowledge and skills are included in the ethics facilitation approach, when responding to HCECs involving conflict among involved parties." "Core Competencies for Healthcare Ethics Consultation," 55.

48 Ibid., 8, footnote 17.

49 Nancy Dubler and Leonard Marcus, *Mediating Bioethical Disputes*, Practical Guide Series (United Hospital Fund, 1994).; Dubler and Liebman, *Bioethics Mediation: A Guide to Shaping Shared Solutions*.

50 *Bioethics Mediation: A Guide to Shaping Shared Solutions*, 1. The fifth reason given is that mediation literature can enrich bioethics literature.

51 Ibid., xv.

52 Ibid.

53 Ibid., xix.

54 Ibid.

55 Efforts are underway, however, including most notably efforts to benchmark clinical ethics consultation and standardize clinical ethics fellowship programs. See The Clinical Ethics Consultation Benchmarking Collaborative, https://

cecbc.net.; Ellen Fox and Jason Adam Wasserman, "Clinical Ethics Fellowship Programs in the United States and Canada: Program Directors' Opinions About Accreditation and Funding," *AJOB Empirical Bioethics* 16, no. 1 (2024): 1–9; Wayne N. Shelton and Bruce D. White, "The Process to Accredit Clinical Ethics Fellowship Programs Should Start Now," *The American Journal of Bioethics* 16, no. 3 (2016): 28–30.

56 Dubler and Liebman, *Bioethics Mediation: A Guide to Shaping Shared Solutions*, xix.

57 Ibid., 21–30.

58 Morreim writes that these principles are "universal," having been endorsed by major organizations such as the International Ombudsman Association's Code of Ethics, the American Arbitration Association, American Bar Association, and Association for Conflict Resolution, based on longstanding agreement and experience regarding the best-functioning mediation. See Morreim, "Mediating in Healthcare's Clinical Setting: Time for a Course Correction," 85–6.

59 Notice that these principles serve the mediation process (the technique's goals), rather than the attainment of goods which are valuable for their own sake.

60 Morreim, "Mediating in Healthcare's Clinical Setting: Time for a Course Correction," 82–3, italics original.

61 Ibid., 89, italics original.

62 Ibid., 84.

63 Ibid., 85.

64 ASBH uses the terminology "principled resolution" to refer to the outcome of CEC: a resolution agreed upon by all parties (ideally) yet also within the bounds of legal and ethical options.

65 Morreim, "Mediating in Healthcare's Clinical Setting: Time for a Course Correction," 105.

66 Morreim isn't the only one to reach this conclusion. ASBH seems to have come to a similar conclusion given how they carve up ethics expertise. See the section below, *A Note on ASBH's Ethics Facilitation Standards*.

67 Dubler and Liebman, *Bioethics Mediation: A Guide to Shaping Shared Solutions.*, 43.

68 Ibid., 44.

69 Ibid.

70 Moyse, *Reading Karl Barth, Interrupting Moral Technique, Transforming Biomedical Ethics*, 105.

71 Jordan Mason, "Techniques of Ordering and the Dynamism of Being: A Critique of Standardized Clinical Ethics Consultation Methods," *HEC Forum* 35 (2022): 8.
72 Dubler and Liebman, *Bioethics Mediation: A Guide to Shaping Shared Solutions*, 59.
73 Ibid., 60., italics added.
74 Ibid., 61.
75 Ibid., 64.
76 Ibid.
77 Ibid., 70.
78 Ibid., 66.
79 The *Core Competencies* claims, "There is general consensus in the field that "ethics facilitation" is the best model for HCEC." They do not offer evidence to support this conclusion. "Core Competencies for Healthcare Ethics Consultation," 6.
80 Ibid., 10.
81 Ibid., 12–13.
82 Legal standards are straightforward, but scholarly literature and bioethical standards are vague, given the lack of consensus about many things in the field.
83 Ibid., 14–16.
84 Ellen Fox et al., *Ethics Consultation: Responding to Ethics Questions in Health Care* (Washington, DC: U.S. Department of Veterans Affairs, 2015).
85 Ibid., 1. Italics original.
86 Ibid., iii.
87 Ibid., 1.
88 Ibid.; A. K. Jha et al., "Effects of the Transformation of the Veterans Affairs Health Care System on the Quality of Care," *New England Journal of Medicine* 348, no. 22 (2003): 2218–27; S. A. Asch et al., "Comparison of Quality of Care for Patients in the Veterans Health Administration and Patients in a National Sample," *Annals of Internal Medicine* 141, no. 12 (2004): 938–45; Catherine Arnst, "The Best Medical Care in the US," *Business Week*, July 17, 2006.
89 The primer states, "Today, every VA medical center has an ethics consultation service, but there's great variability across the VA health care system in terms of the knowledge, skills, and processes brought to bear in performing clinical ethics consultation. Ethics consultation may be the only area in health care in which we allow staff who aren't required to meet clear professional standards, and whose qualifications and expertise can vary greatly, to be so deeply involved in critical, often life-and-death decisions. IntegratedEthics is designed to address

that problem through CASES, a step-by-step approach to ensuring that ethics consultation is of high quality." Fox et al., "Ethics Consultation: Responding to Ethics Questions in Health Care," 6.

90 See Jonathan Moreno, *Deciding Together: Bioethics and Moral Consensus* (Oxford: Oxford University Press, 1995); Tristram Engelhardt, "Credentialing Strategically Ambiguous and Heterogeneous Social Skills: The Emperor without Clothes"; N. Colgrove and K. K. Evans, "The Place for Religious Content in Clinical Ethics Consultations: A Reply to Janet Malek," 31, no. 4 (2019): 305–23.

91 Fox et al., "Ethics Consultation: Responding to Ethics Questions in Health Care," ii. Italics added.

92 L. J. Schneiderman, T. Gilmer, and H. D. Teetzel, "Impact of Ethics Consultations in the Intensive Care Setting: A Randomized, Controlled Trial," *Critical Care Medicine* 28, no. 12 (2000): 3920–4; L. J. Schneiderman et al., "Effect of Ethics Consultations on Nonbeneficial Life-Sustaining Treatments in the Intensive Care Setting: A Randomized Controlled Trial," *JAMA* 290, no. 9 (2003): 1166–72; M. D. Dowdy, C. Robertson, and J. A. Bander, "A Study of Proactive Ethics Consultation for Critically and Terminally Ill Patients with Extended Lengths of Stay," *Critical Care Medicine* 26, no. 11 (1998): 252–9; B. J. Heilicser, D. Meltzer and Mark Siegler, "The Effect of Clinical Medical Ethics Consultation on Healthcare Costs," *J Clin Ethics* 11, no. 1 (2000): 31–8.

93 Fox et al., "Ethics Consultation: Responding to Ethics Questions in Health Care," 1.

94 Ibid., 2.

95 The CASES method builds upon the work of Albert Jonsen, Mark Siegler, and William Winslade, the authors of the Four Boxes method. Readers will likely notice similarities.

96 Fox et al., "Ethics Consultation: Responding to Ethics Questions in Health Care," 27.

97 Ibid., 30.

98 This is, of course, unless the requester is the patient, although it is not clear whether the VA allows patients to make consult requests.

99 Fox et al., "Ethics Consultation: Responding to Ethics Questions in Health Care," 31.

100 The insistence on a concise question reflects the medical specialist consultation process. Consulting with specialist departments like infectious disease or psychiatry requires a narrowing down of the case into a concise question relevant to the consulted department. Whether this is helpful in those contexts is outside the scope of my work. However, when this model is uncritically imported into consultations with ethics, it presents unique problems.

101 This anonymized case really occurred and was described to me by the clinical ethics consultant verbatim as seen here.
102 Fox et al., "Ethics Consultation: Responding to Ethics Questions in Health Care," 35.
103 Ibid., 36.
104 The instruction to carefully distinguish between facts and value judgements diverges significantly from the instructions in Clinical Pragmatism to use both facts and values as equally informative data points for analysis. While both methods place an emphasis on pragmatic problem solving, CASES seems to be more committed to the fact/value distinction, prioritizing facts in the deliberation process.
105 Fox et al., "Ethics Consultation: Responding to Ethics Questions in Health Care," 38.
106 Dubler and Liebman, *Bioethics Mediation: A Guide to Shaping Shared Solutions*.
107 Fox et al., "Ethics Consultation: Responding to Ethics Questions in Health Care," 39.
108 Ibid., 48. The assessment tool to gather feedback can be found at www.ethics.va.gov/IntegratedEthics.
109 Finder and Bliton, *Peer Review, Peer Education, and Modeling in the Practice of Clinical Ethics Consultation: The Zadeh Project*, 7. This book is licensed under the terms of the Creative Commons Attribution 4.0 International License (http://creativecommons.org/licenses/by/4.0/). No changes were made.

4

Richard Zaner's Phenomenological Method

Does truth exist? Is it real or ideal? . . . These primordial questions are surely now superseded by the concerns of philosophy, whether Analytic or Continental. Or have these questions now begun to return?—Catherine Pickstock[1]

In this chapter, I turn my attention to a very different CEC method. Richard Zaner's phenomenological method is quite a bit more procedurally flexible than the others; in fact, Zaner's approach can hardly be considered a standardized technique at all. Rather than attempting to secure high-quality, reliable ethics and demonstrate it to the medical establishment through standardized processes, Zaner maintains the integrity of ethics as a search for the good in the mode of *poiesis*. His method utilizes phenomenological inquiry, a flexible philosophical technique, to grant the ethicist access to the seemingly hidden realities of the crisis from the perspectives of those involved. Then, the ethicist uses her epistemic access to facilitate a moral "encounter," not of her own but between the physician and patient as primary moral agents. Listening, supporting, and asking questions are the main ethical actions. This process is intended primarily to enable the patient's own ethical decision-making, often in ways that defy objective measurement or demonstrability.

Zaner's method is attractive to many philosophically minded ethicists for exactly this reason. Because it rejects procedural ossification and attempts to get close to the patient's reality, Zaner's method solves most of the problems of challenging-forth I've highlighted thus far. Indeed, Zaner's emphasis on "encounter" and his attention to concrete context sounds like it would be a solution to standardization's problems. Zaner gets CEC right in many ways. Yet, in my view, phenomenology still operates within erroneous metaphysical assumptions about the nature of being(s). Phenomenology as a method for

CEC introduces critical difficulties even as it ameliorates others; I will show how phenomenology stops short of revealing goods of and for human being(s). In practice, Zaner's method also risks esotericism, centering the consultant rather than the patient, refusing to acknowledge or engage with intractable disagreement, and failing to offer normative guidance.

Zaner's Phenomenological Method

Background

Zaner's approach to CEC has been articulated in a variety of articles, essays, and books over time. It is hard to distill, and nowhere does he offer a step-by-step explanation of his method, but his distinctive approach can be discerned by a careful reading of his writings. Zaner began writing in the 1960s, his work gradually developing into his characteristic phenomenological bioethics in the 1980s with the publication of well-known works like "Is 'Ethicist' Anything to Call a Philosopher?", *The Context of Self: A Phenomenological Inquiry Using Medicine as a Clue*, and *Ethics and the Clinical Encounter*.[2] Since then, Zaner has been a prolific contributor to the field of bioethics and clinical ethics specifically. He is now professor emeritus at Vanderbilt University Department of Medicine.

Zaner began developing his phenomenological approach to CEC in the midst of larger shifts happening in practical ethics in the late 1980s and early 1990s. At that time, practical ethicists were shifting their focus from content (static theories and principles) to process (methods and goals), partly in an effort to make ethics more relevant and responsive to on-the-ground challenges.[3] Practical relevance seemed nowhere more urgent than in healthcare, where technology was advancing at an alarming rate and ethical challenges were becoming increasingly complex. "It ought to be clear that restricting moral discourse to the formal level of principles, or that of social policy, fails in several ways to be responsive to the real, clinical demands [of cases] . . . When we are in doubt, appeal to principles or policies does not help us decide what to do," Zaner wrote in 1988.[4] The inflexibility, or even irrelevance, of formal ethics principles was a major concern for Zaner, as for other bioethicists; in response to this concern, Zaner began writing about a different kind of clinical ethics. But instead of doubling down on standardized procedures—and making them just as static as theories and principles—to ensure relevance and quality like other ethicists, Zaner opened up clinical ethics to phenomenology.

Clinical ethics must, in order to be helpful, know the facts (both objective and subjective, clinical and experiential) of actual circumstances in their concreteness. Zaner's vision of CEC has firm footing in both the intellectual discipline of philosophical ethics and the real situation, and phenomenology is the bridge between them. Addressing moral crises in medicine, he says, is not a matter of starting from principles or abstract theories and applying them to cases. Rather, because crises arise within concrete clinical situations, their resolution will only be found from within. Efforts at resolving moral crises must attend to the circumstances of each patient and the unique experiential dimensions of the case.[5]

Phenomenology, as a philosophical technique, requires bracketing our existing assumptions, theories, and interpretations, attuning instead to the subject's direct experience of the concrete phenomenon in order to understand what knowledge or actions should be brought to bear. Zaner thus understands a "phenomenology of illness" to be the crucial starting place for accessing the "contextured" reality of clinical cases because the lived experience of illness is the bedrock of all medical moral crises.[6] From this basis, he endeavors to enter into CEC as a philosopher, a medical outsider, using the methods and techniques of phenomenology to listen to patients and begin to draw out their own moral solutions.

But there are obstacles with which to contend. Zaner wants to enter the clinical domain as a philosopher, but medical contexts are driven by a countervailing ethos of efficiency, routine, procedure, and power. He seems to feel this dissonance deeply. Zaner writes in his book *Ethics and the Clinical Encounter* about the danger of being absorbed into the ethos of the hospital and of compromising the integrity of philosophy as a discipline.[7] He worries that ethicists will be co-opted by the *techne*-ical ethos of the medical system, which seems to have borne out in cases where ethics proceduralism rules; if not co-opted, the philosopher "runs the risk of becoming schizophrenic—split between the familiar things of 'home' and the strangeness of medicine. What is at stake is losing professional credibility in both fields."[8] In order to retain philosophical credibility, Zaner remains committed to rejecting standardized procedures and approaching CEC as a medical outsider, although the danger of self-splitting seems to have endured. Zaner may not have fully grasped the extent to which self-splitting hinders his ethics, albeit a different type of self-splitting than the one acknowledged here. I will reinterpret phenomenology's self-splitting in the coming pages.

Despite these dangers, Zaner remains faithful to the tradition of ethical inquiry, with its firmly established concepts of responsibility, responsiveness, and freedom.[9] Zaner concludes his book *Ethics and the Clinical Encounter* with reflections on the nature of moral responsibility and its relation to freedom, reflections which illuminate the virtues of his approach. The Western bioethical tradition is familiar with the prioritization of respect for autonomy—in its simplistic sense, individualistic freedom of choice. But autonomy cannot be a moral foundation for medicine, says Zaner, because we are not essentially remote from others, but are instead *together with* and *alongside* others at every turn. Mutuality and togetherness define human being(s), and thus ground ethical practice.

> The moral order is fundamentally a communal phenomenon. Even though it is clear enough that freedom is in a crucial sense prerequisite for there being moral responsibility, this freedom is not a matter of autonomy but rather a matter of affiliative appealing and responding on behalf of the accidents of birth and circumstance and their "moral chance."[10]

The ethical practice of medicine is thus a *glimpse* into our common humanity and frailty, a *recognition* of that commonness, and then an active *response* aimed at the goods common to us all, which is real freedom. The role of the clinical ethicist is to assist in the relational dynamic by which the medical professional freely responds and becomes responsible to the person who suffers. Our job is to "enable and empower" those on both sides of the professional-patient relationship to maintain their integrities and to increase their capacities for relating with each other.[11]

Restoration, wholeness, self-efficacy, affiliation with the other, integrity, true freedom, moral responsiveness: these are some of the goods at which CEC rightfully aims. What is more, Zaner recognizes that an "encounter" with an ill person can be transformative; it can awaken morality in the physician qua well person.[12] So the ethical medical "encounter" not only serves the integrity and wholeness of the patient, but secondarily of the physician too. Here Zaner is correctly attuned to the participatory element of moral inquiry between the physician and the patient as human beings.

He is also aware that for its own integrity ethics must not copy medicine's efficiency paradigm. An ethics that proves truly morally responsive to the concrete demands of healthcare is an ethics that is *imprecise*. Appealing to Aristotle, who said "precision cannot be expected in the treatment of all subjects alike,"[13] Zaner argues that ethics consists of general rules that apply sometimes but not always. Practical ethics is about prudential decisions on particular points, which is characteristically imprecise. "The agent must consider on each different occasion what the situation demands," said Aristotle.[14] Zaner remains committed to the demands of a responsive ethics, heading off any expectations of straightforward, efficient, or standardized CEC.

Zaner gets a good many things right in his analysis of and vision for CEC. He displays excellent clarity about the purpose and possibility of clinical ethics qua moral inquiry. He tries not to compromise practicality nor theory, but rather to remain faithful to the feedback loop of practical ethics. He avoids the trap of equating quality with uniformity, and of standardizing procedures in order to secure a place for ethics in the medical system. He writes with admirable clarity and emotion about moral responsibility, affiliative appeal, and the ethical response. Perhaps most importantly, he tries to attend to reality and human being(s) as they are: "Any case presents its own set of issues, moral and other. These are context-specific and, as such, require for their identification and delineation an approach and method that are sensitive to what is unique to each case and capable of articulating each in its own terms."[15] Zaner's phenomenology intends to offer epistemological access to the otherwise incomprehensible experience of the other, the vulnerable patient, who Zaner sees as both the subject of the ethical dilemma and the source of its resolution.

Yet Zaner's methodology falls short for exactly the same reason: phenomenology's ontology is one in which beings are separated by a gulf of unknowability. In phenomenological frameworks, only in pure awareness—pre-conceptual experience—do reality and being touch the mind. For phenomenologists, then, the possibility of knowing (for Husserl), ethics (for Levinas), and encounter (for Zaner) hangs on the philosopher's ability to bracket her preconceived ideas and theories, which hinder concrete awareness. Said another way, being(s) are radically unknowable to each other except through an escape from the mind's *enframing* effects. While Zaner appeals in his writing to mutuality and togetherness, the moral encounter that Zaner describes as resulting from bracketing is subtly but crucially different from the encounter that is integral to the participatory bringing-forth of human goods; Zaner's encounter is something that can only be facilitated by an ethicist who has set aside her thoughts, ideas, training—in many ways, her *self*. We must ask ourselves, then, whether Zaner's intention of a CEC with mutuality, recognition, responsiveness, affiliative appealing, etc., can be realized within this system.

Methodology

As is clear by now, Zaner's intention, shared by the wider clinical ethics community, is that CEC should be responsive to the actual contexts in which medical moral crises occur. For Zaner, this responsiveness and relevance constitutes quality CEC, a truly practical ethics. The development of his approach to CEC thus rests on the following three theses: (1) The work of ethics requires strict focus on the specific *situational definition* of each involved person; (2) Moral issues are presented solely *within the contexts* of their actual occurrence; and (3) The situational participants are the *principal resources* for the resolution of the moral issues presented.[16] What could this possibly mean for CEC methodology? In other words, what is there for the ethicist to *do*?

Thesis one brings Zaner to the conclusion that "The problems presented by a case are the problems of those whose case it is, just as are the alternatives, decisions, and aftermaths."[17] Ethicists should understand themselves as acting on behalf of the situational participants, each of whom has their own story about the case, its problems and possibilities, options, and decision points. The ethicist must thus start the CEC process by getting into the experience and interpretation of each participant. CECs are fundamentally observers.[18] In fact, while Zaner is wary of rules for CEC, one of his two "rules of method" is that "in-person interactions with situational participants are a far better source of evidence for description, interpretation, and thematic judgements than secondhand reports."[19]

Thesis two leads to complementary criteria: CECs must be focused on the phenomenon of everyday discourse between patients and their medical practitioners, as well as attentive awareness to the physical, historical, and cultural setting in which the discourse takes place.[20] Stuart Finder and Mark Bliton, students of Zaner's, write, "the clinical and moral work of clinical ethics consultation is primarily communicative, involving many varied forms of telling and listening which thereby elicit additional repetitions, including written forms, to establish clearly, to the extent possible, what is morally relevant."[21] They are onto something important when they recognize the "varied forms" of telling and listening, and the need for multiple repetitions of communication in order to gain moral insight. They are intuitively understanding the requirements of ethics in a world that consists of non-identical repetitions. Zaner poignantly explains his second and final rule of method:

> Every life is linguistically inexhaustible, there is always a richer tale to be told that can never be wholly captured in words. . . . Interpretation is essentially limited by all that which spills out beyond out words; there is always more to be told, no matter how much we know, hence what is said is always on this side of definitive or certain.[22]

We cannot capture being(s) in words because being(s) always exceed our knowledge; this existential humility is the stance from which wise practical ethicists have learned to approach dilemmas.

Lastly, because of thesis three, CEC should look to the people involved in the case (the patient, family, physicians, nurses, social workers, consulting physicians, etc.) to resource the solution. The problem is theirs, they must live with the consequences, so they must make the decision.[23] Ethicists' work at the decision-making stage is to assist patients (and sometimes surrogates or family members on patients' behalf) in the elucidation of their beliefs and values, the appreciation of what their circumstances mean for them, and the consideration of the best way forward.[24] But all participants, leaving aside the ethicist, have valuable insight to offer in this process.

Not formulated into specific steps per se, Zaner's method loosely follows this path: *observe* the situation from the perspective of those involved, *listen* to those involved using a phenomenological lens, *pay attention* to the setting and context in which your listening occurs, and *empower* participants to find their own solution. "Enablement," or empowerment, is a central methodological concept in his approach. Empowering ethics work endeavors to help people find their own resources for dealing with difficult situations, offering them support and validation, clarity, and focus.[25]

Zaner's method is a wonderful representation of phenomenology, and it reflects normative stances on the nature of good decision-making, but it carries little normative bioethical content into the CEC process. Because Zaner's CEC is so thoroughly focused on the participants (patient, family, care team, etc.) and the communication between them—as opposed to, say, normative ethical determinations or decisions, which are bracketed out—he calls his approach "clinical-liaison ethics." He stands *between* the medical team and the patient/family, both correcting communication errors and elucidating (but not necessarily resolving) deeper values that may be in conflict.[26]

While they differ in many respects, in this way Zaner's approach and Bioethics Mediation are alike. They both approach CEC as if ethicists are more or less neutral parties, liaisons between the "real" participants who should be making decisions. Clinical liaison work involves probing and interpreting issues, mapping out and testing strategies, assisting decision-making, and supporting the aftermath—but not recommending an ethical decision. Normative guides and boundaries are even more lacking in Zaner's CEC than in Bioethics Mediation because phenomenology requires they be intentionally sidelined in order to understand the situation. The foreseeable problems with such an approach may be obvious, but I will highlight two here. First, the patient/surrogate may make a decision that is ethically unsupportable, and Zaner does not clarify what the ethicist should do in such a case. If the patient/surrogate is enabled and supported in *any* decision they make, Zaner's method becomes proceduralism in another guise, and the technique legitimizes the (potentially bad) outcome yet again. Lack of normative recommendations from the ethicist can also leave participants sincerely confused. If the ethics consult goes beyond simple miscommunication or lack of support and presents as a situation with competing goods, Zaner's method is ill-equipped to help resolve it. Reflecting on a phenomenological CEC process, Andrea Frolic and Susan Rubin write,

> While it's not the job of the ethics consultant to be prescriptive or determinative, in our view there is an inescapably normative dimension to the work. Our focus is on the "ought" questions. We're not there to simply name and comment on what is. Or to be passive observers. Or even to offer a supportive presence. We ought to have something unique and value added to contribute. And that contribution shouldn't be based simply on our ability to play well with others or make people feel safe, comfortable, and supported. It should be grounded in the discipline of ethics and should contribute something recognizably different and valuable to the equation.[27]

While Zaner's method theoretically unites ethical theory with practice, this unity begins to come apart as the method is deployed. Practice becomes all-consuming, and ethical content, principles, and norms never seem to resurface. If no recommendation is made and no content brought to bear, as seems to be the case at least the majority of the time in Zaner's method, it must be asked whether this approach remains "ethics."

Second, the liaison work for which Zaner's method calls requires the ethicist to attempt a type of self-erasure. This element is a consequence of phenomenology's ontological assumptions, as noted above, that persons are radically inaccessible to each other, something only potentially ameliorated by precise "bracketing" of parts of the self that would hold us back from pure experience, the site of knowing. This process seems to truly be a self-splitting, although of a different type than the philosopher-medical professional self-splitting acknowledged by Zaner. Bracketing creates two selves in the ethicist: the self that observes without concepts, and the self that apprehends and measures truth. Self-splitting, successful or not, actually prevents a reciprocal ethical encounter from occurring between the ethicist and CEC participants because the integrated self is not brought to bear—parts of the self are erased.

Additionally, while it may intuitively seem that an ethicist's attempt at self-erasure would center the patient and the physician, whom Zaner believes are the real subjects of the ethical process, in practice an ethicist's attempt at self-erasure can appear to have the opposite effect. Phenomenological CEC can appear to be all about the ethicist and his correct execution of phenomenological methodology. In fact, CEC thus framed is impossible unless done Zaner's way. To understand these concerns more fully, let's dive deeper into the theoretical issues with this method.

Foucault's Critique of Phenomenology and Other Kantian Philosophies

Phenomenology does not fall to the standardization critique I leveled against the other methods. Yet, there are other reasons why it is not the solution to practical ethics' questions of technique. Michel Foucault, in his critique of the human sciences, offers a way to understand the theoretical problems inherent in phenomenology. Foucault is a complex figure; it is hard to place his work within any particular discipline. He touches on social science, politics, and medicine from both historical/genealogical and philosophical lenses. As Jeffrey P. Bishop points out, Foucault is usually considered a philosopher by historians and a historian by philosophers.[28] He described himself as a historian of thought or a historian of problematizations.[29] Either way, it has been suggested that Foucault's organizing question could be stated: How is it possible to have true knowledge, and what are the necessary conditions of that knowledge?[30] Foucault's organizing question makes sense when we consider that he is Kantian. Kant problematizes "true knowledge" by insisting that there is no way for us to verify whether our mental concepts of things actually correspond to things in themselves. How then are we to gain knowledge? How are we to trust it? Foucault's work takes up these questions and attempts to solve some of the problems created by Kant. While he is quite successful at diagnosing problems of modern thought, he is less adept at offering solutions; I will use his work only to lead us to the source of phenomenology's insufficiencies for CEC.[31]

To gain insight into phenomenology's mistaken assumptions, Foucault follows the genealogy of thought that made phenomenology possible and even necessary. In Classical thought, things were understood to be representations of the transcendent. This is often referred to as the *analogia entis*—the analogy of being, which I described in Chapter 2. As a reminder, in the *analogia entis*, things (*res*) were understood as participating in being (*ens*) through their forms. According to John Milbank, "One can retrospectively narrate Plato's and Aristotle's writings as a groping towards the linking of universal with particular, as also the individual with the whole, the family with the city, contemplation with practice."[32] Mutual participation implied these linkages. Importantly, this participatory ontology grounded empirical knowledge and analysis: we can trust empirical knowledge of particulars because our intellect participates in *ens*, and thus in the transcendentals (Goodness, Truth, and Beauty). Foucault describes this as the Classical "correlation" between a metaphysics of representation of the transcendent and an analysis of finite beings.[33] Within such a system, finitude (the particular; *res*) referred back to the infinite (the universal; *ens*), avoiding the need to ground knowledge from within the realm of finitude with all of its attendant theoretical pitfalls. The particular corresponded with the universal, or as Foucault writes, there was a middle ground between the "positivist" and the "eschatological" which has not since been achieved.

Then came a change in the metaphysical system. As I described in Chapter 2, Scotus and Ockham set off a new type of ontological thinking that immanentized being. Called the "univocity of being," this ontology rejected similitudes in nature, rejected the participatory grounding of knowledge, and created an epistemological problem that would pave the way for Kant. If *res* no longer participate in *ens*, how can we be sure we can access reality? How can we trust the human mind to apprehend things in themselves? Isn't all human knowledge then conditional, created, untrustworthy? As Foucault puts it, because the human mind can hardly be trusted to transcend itself, finitude is now in "an interminable cross-reference with itself."[34]

Modern philosophy has been dealing with these questions ever since. In part, says Foucault, the effort to preserve human knowledge has brought us to theoretical dualisms that are in some sense arbitrary. In any case, they are problematic. In the modern era, the human sciences operate under three such arbitrary theoretical divisions of knowledge as a result of Kantian philosophy. These include 1) rudimentary and emergent knowledge vs. stable and definitive knowledge, 2) illusion vs. verifiable knowledge, and 3) empirical vs. transcendental truth.[35] These divisions make possible certain types of study by grounding knowledge, giving it opposing categories within which to situate itself. The first and second have to do with studying the natural and historical conditions of knowledge, respectively. The third, though, has to do with the human being herself as knower.

Because the human sciences have the human being for both their subject *and* their object, they require the human to be both the knower and the known. The human is both *experiencing* phenomena and *making sense of* herself experiencing that phenomena—simultaneously apprehending both subjective and objective forms of knowledge. In other words, the human is dualistically divided between the empirical mind (observing reality) and the transcendental mind (organizing/interpreting what is observed and supposedly attuning to the Good, the True, and the Beautiful). In Kant's *Anthropology from a Practical Point of View*, Foucault finds that "there is an ambivalence between the transcendental constituting subject and the already constituted object."[36] This tension within the self is what Foucault terms the "empirico-transcendental doublet:" "For the threshold of our modernity is situated not by the attempt to apply objective methods to the study of man, but rather by the constitution of an empirico-transcendental doublet which was called *man*."[37] Foucault says that philosophy in the wake of Kant has searched for a discourse that allows both to remain in tension, so that there can exist both the empirically known (immanent) and also the True (transcendent). This discourse is phenomenology—the study of experience.

Phenomenology theoretically allows for a communication between the individual body and wider culture, between nature and history, writes Foucault. It attempts to ground epistemological knowledge *and* restore transcendental knowledge (the Good, the True, and the Beautiful) by appealing to pure bodily experience as the site of both types of knowledge. Put differently, the moment of pre-cognitive bodily experience is thought to both ground our knowledge of concrete situations—what is—*and* our knowledge of ethics—what should be. But Foucault discerns the futility of this appeal:

> This analysis seeks to articulate the possible objectivity of a knowledge of nature upon the original experience of which the body provides an outline. . . . It is doing no more, then, than fulfilling with greater care the hasty demands laid down when the attempt was made to make the empirical, in man, stand for the transcendental.[38]

Phenomenology fulfills the demands of modern thinking by participating in two dualisms, one ontological and one epistemological. Ontologically, the human must be both an empirical, embodied, emotive person *in* the "real world" and a transcendent, universal something (the ego, reason, the soul, etc.) which accesses something *beyond* the "real world" and which keeps the embodied person in check. Epistemologically, the knowledge ascertained by this human is divided between that of the knowing subject and that of the object of study. The human is thus an active subject and a passive object of variegated knowledge.

This type of thinking is evident in Zaner's approach to CEC. His method requires a separation within the ethicist between her theoretical, "universal" knowledge of ethics and theories and her bodily experience of the concrete phenomenon. Zaner unwittingly rehearses the empirico-transcendental doublet in his search to ground knowledge. As Foucault warns, phenomenological inquiry cannot actually unite the two, and so usually turns merely to the empirical: "The phenomenological project continually resolves itself, before our eyes, into a description—empirical despite itself—of actual experience."[39] Even more troubling for our purposes, the possibility of morality is closed by this empirical bent. "For modern thought, no morality is possible,"[40] writes Foucault. Indeed we see this lack of normativity playing out in Zaner's method; for all its talk about the possibility of a moral transformation, it stops short of being able to rise above empirical description.

While Foucault is correct that phenomenology usually privileges the empirical and loses the normative, there is a sense in which Zaner reacts by pulling the transcendental-self back into his CEC method. This transcendental-self steps into the empirical-self's interactions with CEC participants by helping them describe, through repetition and revision, their story of events in a cohesive and coherent way. Contrary to what he might wish or claim, Zaner's transcendental-self is not erased, but re-emerges as the one helping physicians, patients, families, nurses, etc., curate a description of the medical realities of the case, along with their roles, grievances, desires, values, etc. The participants' descriptions come to constitute them as objects in a particular narration, and this process turns Zaner into the creator of the objects' self-understanding. This transcendental position is in a sense god-like because it is a position above or outside the participants' positions, granting Zaner critical distance. He is not entangled in the multiplicitous narratives as a morally implicated subject; he is the arbiter, the narrator of truth.

Of course, all of this self-splitting and self-erasure sounds quite theoretical and removed from the reality of what is occurring in CEC—because it is. The empirico-transcendental doublet and its required self-erasure are not possible because the self cannot be erased or split. In fact, the belief that it can be is a work of the theoretical mind. Zaner's desire to unite the concrete and the theoretical is shared by all practical ethicists, but his method instead enacts a sort of deception. The removed narrating and constituting work of his method runs the risk of being an exertion of authority, an exertion of the power of the supposed transcendental position.

As a Kantian, Foucault recognizes both the need to ground true knowledge and the problems that these resulting dualisms raise in approaches like phenomenology. He searches for a way to resolve the difficulties while avoiding reducing everything to the transcendental—and avoiding rethinking Kant. But according to Bishop, Foucault never solves the problem of the empirico-transcendental doublet seen in phenomenology and other Kantian philosophies.[41] Foucault is clear that a return to "actual experience" in phenomenology will not resolve the doublet, but will rather offer it "confirmation by giving [it] roots;"[42] yet he does not say where we go from here. Could it be that the problem of knowledge cannot be solved without a rethinking of Kant's dualisms? Could it be that the only solution is a participatory ontology?

Phenomenology's Revealing and Concealing

Zaner's CEC method utilizes the methodology of phenomenology to help resolve moral dilemmas in the complex world of medicine. Because Zaner re-situates CEC in the domain of practical ethics, his understanding of ethics expertise is less technocratic than the other methods, and he in fact correctly describes the phenomenon of moral crisis. As all techniques do, Zaner's method both reveals and conceals aspects of reality to allow the ethicist to work with a case in a productive way. It reveals to the ethicist a cacophony of narratives about the conflict or problem by coaxing out into the open each participant's perspective, likely offering a fuller picture of the problem than other methods. It reveals to the participants, through the ethicist's reflective listening, what interests and values may be undergirding their positions. To patients in crisis especially, it may reveal what matters most to them, what remains consistent as they talk through the dilemma again and again. It may reveal space for agreement or for compromise, or even for compassion and transformation. Certainly, Zaner's method offers a possibility of these positive revelations. Yet because the method places the ethicist in the god-like position of constituting the participants as certain kinds of objects within a certain kind of narrative, it carries the potential for the wielding of authority. It removes the ethicist from her implicated position and places her instead in a powerful transcendental place. As it turns out, phenomenology also impedes an ethicist's encounter with being(s) and their good.

While it may reveal in positive or negative ways, this method also must conceal. It conceals parts of the ethicist that may hinder her epistemic deference to other participants. It conceals the moral responsibility of the ethicist to keep participants within certain bounds (i.e., those of institutional policy, legality, and morality). It conceals parts of the ethicist so that they appear split or erased, making an encounter with being(s) impossible. Its revealing/concealing action is perhaps more subtle than the other methods and closer to that which is appropriate for practical ethics. Yet its concealing points to deeper problems with the way this method conceives of ethics in practical settings.

Like the other CEC techniques, Zaner's phenomenological method functions as an *ersatz* liturgy: it is an embodied practice fueled by a moral imaginary of the good life. As we participate in this *ersatz* liturgy, it forms our identities and governs our actions. Like a religious liturgy, it has political, formational, and affective dimensions. Zaner's method ritually defines the ethicist as a neutral facilitator, someone quite removed, rather than a morally implicated normative guide. As the one conducting and bringing to completion the *ersatz* liturgy of phenomenological CEC, the ethicist stands in a god-like position. In part, this serves to protect the ethicist from the institutional and disciplinary power of the hospital; the ethicist is merely listening, merely reflecting and observing, never capable of causing harm. We know cognitively this isn't true, that ethicists are capable of great harm, but liturgical action works affectively and bodily to convince us otherwise. The technique focuses instead on the agency of the patient and the doctor; it isolates the physician-patient dyad and attempts to erase the influence of the ethicist on that dyad.[43] The ethicist can remain the philosopher, the patient can remain the ill person, the physician can remain the healer, and the political life of the institution goes uninterrupted.

I have also shown that Zaner's phenomenological method operates within hidden dualisms which undermine his hope for a responsive and responsible CEC. Phenomenology assumes that knowledge of the good can only be attained through a kind of self-splitting, the empirico-transcendental doublet, through which the ethicist attempts to unite the concrete situation with the Good, True, and Beautiful. It turns out, however, that this doublet no more grounds ethical knowledge than any other technique of secular reason, because the human mind remains in cross-reference with itself.[44] Zaner's lack of overt normativity in active patient cases reflects phenomenology's failure to connect the particular to the universal, the person with the transcendent. But of course, there are covert and subtle forms of normativity inherent in Zaner's narrations for/with/to the participants of "what is going on," participants who are now objects of the ethical gaze. In the end, this method fails for practical ethics.

I agree with Zaner on a great many things, including that a responsive ethics must be accountable for its deliberations and recommendations. "Ethical deliberations here, with real people facing very real moral dilemmas and problems, must be accountable. *A responsive ethics must be a responsible ethics*—responsible for being well informed and responsible both to the providers and to the patients and their families,"[45] he writes. But how can we manage such an ethics in healthcare, given that even phenomenology fails? In Part II, I will begin to answer this question by returning again to the question of being. I will continue to show how practical ethics, a search for the good in concrete circumstances, is a process inseparable from metaphysics. I will argue that the Christian liturgy is the technique *par excellence* for the bringing forth of being(s) and their good, and for interrupting the power and control operative in our existing CEC methods.

Notes

1. Catherine Pickstock, *Aspects of Truth: A New Religious Metaphysics* (Cambridge: Cambridge University Press, 2020), 1. Copyright Catherine Pickstock 2020. Reproduced with permission of The Licensor through PLSclear.
2. Richard Zaner, "Is 'Ethicist' Anything to Call a Philosopher?," *Human Studies* 7 (1984): 71–90; *The Context of Self: A Phenomenological Inquiry Using Medicine as a Clue* (Athens, OH: Ohio University Press, 1981).; Richard M. Zaner, *Ethics and the Clinical Encounter* (Englewood Cliffs, NJ: Prentice Hall, 1988).
3. There were other reasons, too. Importantly, a focus on process helps to secure vestiges of normativity in the secular (morally contested) spaces where practical ethics occurs, including medicine. Normativity can be baked into techniques in ways that seem less contestable than theories and metaphysical systems. Some nonreligious ethicists, such as Abram Brummett, are also beginning to notice the normativity baked into procedural bioethics, identify its problematic nature, and respond with a call to revive metaphysical analysis. See Abram Brummett, "Secular Clinical Ethicists Should Not Be Neutral toward All Religious Beliefs: An Argument for a Moral-Metaphysical Proceduralism," *The American Journal of Bioethics* 21, no. 6 (2021): 5–16; "Whose Harm? Which Metaphysic?," *Theoretical Medicine and Bioethics* 40, no. 1 (2019): 43–61; Abram Brummett and Jason T. Eberl, "The Many Metaphysical Commitments of Secular Clinical Ethics: Expanding the Argument for a Moral-Metaphysical Proceduralism," *Bioethics* 36, no. 7 (2022): 783–93.

4 Zaner, *Ethics and the Clinical Encounter*, 26–7.
5 Ibid.
6 Ibid., 53–91.
7 Ibid., 8–9.
8 Ibid., 9.
9 Ethicists and theologians (including Aristotle, Aquinas, Karl Barth, Dietrich Bonhoeffer, James Keenan, James Bretzke, and Martin Buber, to name a few) have long noted that freedom is a prerequisite for responsibility and that responsiveness is an important element of moral action. These concepts have special meaning for Christian ethicists, who often situate ethical action as a response to the gift, revelation, or salvation of Christ, which is the origin of human freedom.
10 Zaner, *Ethics and the Clinical Encounter*, 310.
11 Ibid., 319–20.
12 Ibid., 305.
13 Aristotle, *The Nicomachean Ethics of Aristotle*, Part 1, Section 3.
14 Ibid., Part 2, Section 3.
15 Zaner, *Ethics and the Clinical Encounter*, 242.
16 Ibid., 242–8, italics added.
17 Ibid., 243.
18 Ibid.
19 Ibid., 269–70.
20 Ibid., 245.
21 Finder and Bliton, *Peer Review, Peer Education, and Modeling in the Practice of Clinical Ethics Consultation: The Zadeh Project.*, 2. This book is licensed under the terms of the Creative Commons Attribution 4.0 International License (http://creativecommons.org/licenses/by/4.0/). No changes were made.
22 Zaner, *Ethics and the Clinical Encounter*, 272.
23 Ibid., 248.
24 Finder and Bliton, *Peer Review, Peer Education, and Modeling in the Practice of Clinical Ethics Consultation: The Zadeh Project*, 3.
25 Zaner, *Ethics and the Clinical Encounter*, 249.
26 Ibid., 244.
27 Frolic and Rubin, "Critical Self-Reflection as Moral Practice: A Collaborative Meditation on Peer Review in Ethics Consultation," 51.

28 Jeffrey P. Bishop, *The Anticipatory Corpse* (Notre Dame, IN: University of Notre Dame Press, 2011), 28.
29 Ibid.
30 Ibid., 29.
31 Ibid., 23.
32 John Milbank, *Theology and Social Theory: Beyond Secular Reason*, 2nd ed. (Malden, MA: Blackwell Publishing, 2006), 331.
33 Michel Foucault, *The Order of Things: An Archaeology of the Human Sciences* (New York: Vintage Books, 1970), 317.
34 Ibid., 318.
35 For an interesting discussion on the eventual fallout of these dualisms (and attempted solutions) in the social sciences today, see Jason Ananda Josephson-Storm, *Metamodernism: The Future of Theory* (Chicago, IL: University of Chicago Press, 2021).
36 Bishop, *The Anticipatory Corpse*, 30.
37 Foucault, *The Order of Things: An Archaeology of the Human Sciences*, 319.
38 Ibid., 321.
39 Ibid., 326.
40 Ibid., 328.
41 Bishop, *The Anticipatory Corpse*, 36.
42 Foucault, *The Order of Things: An Archaeology of the Human Sciences*, 322.
43 Interestingly, Zaner does acknowledge that the one-to-one physician-patient relationship is mainly "the stuff of nostalgia," and that medical practice is always a web of relations. However, his method is built upon the dyad nonetheless. See Zaner, *Ethics and the Clinical Encounter*, 19–20.
44 For a more thorough critique of secular reason in ethics, see especially chapter 11 of Milbank, *Theology and Social Theory: Beyond Secular Reason*.
45 Zaner, *Ethics and the Clinical Encounter*, 28.

Interlude

What Kind of Doing Is Clinical Ethics Consultation?

So then deliberation takes place in such matters as are under general laws, but still uncertain how in any given case they will issue.—Aristotle[1]

An ethics consult request comes through the electronic medical record early on a Friday morning. The consult notes contain a callback name (Dr. Moore), phone number, and a simple note: "Patient delusional, refusing surgery, wants to leave against medical advice, no family members." The ethicist begins her chart review, noting that the 27-year-old patient was admitted 7 days prior for active hallucinations and delusions as well as severe skin infection. The wound care team has recommended surgery on the infected area, but the patient has refused, saying, "The surgeons are working for the mafia from Mars, and they want to remove all the water from my body." No family or friends have been located. Until today, the patient has been content to stay in the hospital as long as he is provided with extra blankets and food, but now he is telling the nursing staff he intends to leave.

After reviewing the chart, the ethicist calls Dr. Moore back for more information and invites her to describe her moral concerns. Dr. Moore articulates concern that she is not equipped to provide the patient with the psychiatric care he needs, concern about the potential for additional harm if the patient leaves the hospital, and uncertainty regarding the permissibility of restraining the patient for surgery. The ethicist affirms Dr. Moore's concerns and discloses her initial ethical thinking on these points but says she will need to call other members of the care team, especially social work and wound care, and see the patient herself before getting back to her with recommendations. Dr. Moore reluctantly agrees and urges the ethicist to work quickly.

The ethicist gathers her knowledge of the legal and policy requirements for psychiatric holds, decision-making without a surrogate, restraints, and patient elopement. She begins to write down the goods at stake for the patient, taking cues from her conversations with members of the medical team. Upon meeting the patient, she gets a sense of the severity of his delusions and the level of risk he might be undertaking if he were to elope from the hospital. She contacts key members of the medical team once more, this time thinking out loud about possible courses of action and how the patient might respond. During this process, the ethicist begins to articulate moral boundaries, such as "restraining the patient is not ethically supportable in this case." As the team discusses the situation, next steps begin to emerge. Dr. Moore is able to convince the patient to stay for one more night (with food, blankets, and extra desserts) so they can arrange for transfer to an accepting psychiatric facility. In the meantime, the nurse most known for her ability to soften patients offers to clean the patient's wound, which he allows, even though he continues to refuse surgery. The ethicist writes a chart note documenting her conversations, ethical and legal boundaries, and ethical recommendations for next steps. The chart note does not resolve the tension between competing goods or offer clean answers to discrete ethics questions (indeed no formulaic "ethics questions" were posed), but offers the team a unifying narrative of the steps taken to ensure compassionate and ethical care for their vulnerable patient.

In Part I we covered a lot of philosophical ground, and through that lens, interrogated the five major CEC methods. We found that standardized methods do in fact blind us to the aspects of reality that they are not set up to reveal. This blinding to certain aspects of reality leads to various downstream problems in CEC, such as intolerance of irreconcilable disagreement, manipulation and the use of procedural power, or lack of normativity. Because our techniques are largely borrowed from other disciplines (standardized techniques are not native to practical ethics), they reveal and conceal what is necessary for those pursuits rather than our own, leading to confusion about what exactly clinical ethics is or should be doing. Downstream problems will continue to haunt our field as long as we attempt to create standardized techniques for CEC. So, we saw that in order for clinical ethics to be responsive to real situations, accommodating of diversity and disagreement, and to lead us toward the true and the good, CEC techniques must allow for an encounter with being(s) by eschewing standardization.

But eschewing standardization alone is not enough; as a careful analysis of Zaner's phenomenological method shows, nonstandardized CEC techniques can still be predicated upon ontological commitments that impede encounter. An encounter is a reciprocal activity, an activity wherein that which is acted upon acts upon the actor: an activity in which the ethicist is *implicated*. Ethicists are not primarily technicians of method, yet ethicists are not primarily removed, neutral observers or mediators either. Even phenomenology—which tries to attend to being(s) in themselves—fails to properly understand the relational nature of being(s), leading phenomenologists to incorrectly describe the activity of CEC, still stuck in the Kantian divide between our minds and reality. So what is the answer? To reject techniques outright would make clinical ethics an ad hoc, relativized activity with the potential to inflict great harm through force at one extreme, or lose all normative value at the other. Is there a way to perform CEC that avoids the traps of standardization and of separation that attunes us to the discernment of concrete goods in particular circumstances? How can we build and evaluate such techniques?

In the chapters that follow, I will offer an emphatic "yes" to the first question and concrete suggestions for the second. But we are not quite at the building stage yet; in order for practical ethicists to develop techniques that enable a search for the good in concrete circumstances, we need to better understand what our work *is*, why we are doing it, and how we will know if we are successful.[2] I have already reflected on the latter question, although briefly; next, I will address the former two questions at some length.

I have identified CEC as a kind of "doing" firmly situated within the family of endeavors called practical ethics. I have appealed to Dennis Thompson's definition of practical ethics as not simply applied ethics (often thought of as bodies of ethical knowledge about certain domains), but more fundamentally an approach by which we allow the concrete realities of these practical contexts to revise our ethical principles and vice versa, in a circular process of continued adjustment and correction.[3] This description of our task, which I take to be vitally important, conjures the mental image of a feedback loop rather than a one-directional vector toward a goal. Relatedly, I have suggested that techniques used in practical ethics ought to be in the mode of *poiesis*, bringing forth goods rather than challenging forth solutions. While I suspect many clinical ethicists would agree with the description of their work as a type of practical ethics, a feedback loop between theory and practice requiring flexible techniques, it is also clear that many clinical ethicists utilize methods, or are taught to utilize methods, or are increasingly expected by ASBH and professional standards to utilize methods, that resemble a vector aiming toward a recommendation in an efficient and reliable manner, such as those methods analyzed in Chapter 3. This mismatch may reflect many factors: time limitations, institutional demands, educational failings, pressures from medical professionals, or other logistical hurdles. Yet even more saliently, this mismatch is likely deeply rooted in an internal debate in the field of clinical ethics about what exactly we are doing when we respond to a consultation request. Based on the historical development of the field and relevant literature about things like ethics expertise, justification, competencies, credentialing, and the like, it is reasonable to conclude that this internal debate or dissensus looms quite large. In fact, the question "what are we doing in CEC?" is one that my colleagues and I regularly ask each other, even those of us who are actively engaged in the professional work of CEC, have a PhD in health care ethics, and are HEC-C certified. This overriding question, which George Agich puts rather succinctly as "what kind of doing is clinical ethics?"[4] has great bearing on the methods and techniques we judge as acceptable. In fact, questions of method and technique nest inside this broader question, so it will be helpful to review my claims about the doing of CEC at this juncture.

Practical ethics is concerned with the good of/for being(s). Because being(s) consist of non-identical repetitions, each being manifesting itself in unique ways in space/time, we know that the good of/for being(s) is contextual; it cannot be known in an abstract sense in advance of an encounter with the particular being(s). For example, think back to the case study at the beginning of this section. Even though the ethicist knows the legal and policy requirements for inpatient psychiatric placement, restraints, treatment over objection, and decision-making in the absence of a surrogate decision maker, she could not have known in advance what was good for this patient refusing surgery. Indeed, beyond law and policy, even though the ethicist is the resident expert on the bioethics literature regarding these situations—arguments for and against restraints for patients who refuse care, etc.—she could not know what to recommend until she had encountered the complexities and nuances of this particular patient's case. The good for being(s) cannot be known abstractly, but only in context.

Yet good is also connected to the Good, a transcendental, which carries normative implications that will be true across contexts and manifestations of being, as all being is participating in God. The ethicist must know, in general, when it is and is not ethically justifiable to perform surgery on someone against their will, i.e. when it is justifiable to use force against another for their own good. There are things we can and should say about the use of force against other living beings in general. So practical ethics is a kind of meeting between the concrete and the transcendental; it is an activity which requires holding both the contextual, unpredictable, emergent concrete situation *and* the eternally true, which we can only know in part, and our knowledge of which we will always be fallible and provisional. CEC as a practical ethical endeavor, then, must be something more than technical skill *and* more than theoretical knowledge. It must be a reflective practice, wherein ethicists both attune themselves to an encounter with reality and their provisional understanding of ethical theory.

Practical ethics is a feedback loop, then, but one that requires a certain attentiveness to what exceeds our gaze on each side. It's a moral activity that is reflective and reflexive, and done in participation with others. It is immediately evident in the practice of clinical ethics that an ethicist cannot make good recommendations alone. She must involve herself in the moral struggling of the primary decision-makers and medical professionals, the agents who carry out (or not) her recommendations. The ethicist, then, is both striving for the good and facilitating the striving of others for the good.

The grammatical concept of the "middle voice" helps capture more clearly what I mean. In the middle voice, the subject both performs (as the agent) and receives (as the direct object) the action of the verb, i.e. "he stretches" or "the casserole bakes." When a person stretches, are they the one stretching or the one being stretched? The middle voice *transcends* the duality of active vs. passive, and of inside vs. outside the self. In fact, the middle voice refuses to distinguish between the subject and the object of an action. Quite common in ancient Indo-European languages, modern English retains only pieces of the middle voice, sometimes in intransitive verbs or with the assistance of a reflexive pronoun. Yet modern English obscures the radical meaning of the middle voice if it relegates it only to the reflexive. It is not simply that the subject performs a process on/within himself (reflexively); it's about *shared agency* rather than an inward or reflexive directionality.[5]

As Jan Gonda describes, in the middle voice, agency is shared in such a way that it can also be said to be *suppressed*: the verb is grammatically active but semantically passive, agency being of little importance to the meaning conveyed because in fact agency is always shared.[6] The middle voice also, then, denotes a relationality, a participation, between the noun and the verb, or between the noun and other nouns. In ancient usage, the middle voice was often used in the future tense; Gonda believes future usage of the middle voice was connected to the tendency to use imprecise terms for the future since the future is always uncertain. The middle voice allows the speaker to be reserved in their claims about what will happen in the future, both what will happen to themselves and to other people, and what will happen as a result of themselves and other people.[8]

The concept of the middle voice has been taken up by continental and postmodern philosophers to articulate the troubling of the categories of agency and certainty, and the displacement of the subject.[9] It has been used in attempts to reconcile the falsely separated categories of inside (imaginary) and outside (real), the Kantian legacy.[10] It has been described by Jacques Derrida as a voice that indicates interlacing, such as a stitching up of two sides of fabric, or a rhythmic movement, an oscillation.[11] The middle voice offers a way to think beyond our modern English-speaking conceptual and linguistic framework of subject-object dualities. It is not a metaphor, but a reality of being, which has been distorted by our contemporary dualistic thinking. The middle voice expresses the ontological truth that life is always participatory. In acting, I am acted upon; in deploying a technique, it is deployed also upon me; in giving to another I receive; in coming into being, I bring into being two parents.

I would like to suggest that CEC is rightly a middle-voice activity. In practical ethics, a true middle voice ought to be enacted: our ego as subject decentered and our agential gaze disrupted and transformed. We ought to engage in a different kind of seeing, open and reciprocal, which might be called beholding. We should be shown to be interconnected and contingent with the rest of creation, rather than independently efficacious. Our work and its effects on us and others are neither entirely active nor entirely passive; the active/passive distinction is muddied, and this disruption of the usual direction of agency leads to new relational possibilities. Communion or relation is recognized as an ontological concept, as all things are in constant relation and in constant motion out from themselves, mirroring Derrida's interlacing and oscillation. Importantly, the approach to goodness and truth is not completed by our own power. We must look beyond ourselves, aware of the limits of our knowing, constantly re-beginning the search lest we believe it were a matter of correctly deploying a certain technique. We must be eminently aware of the possibility of our own failure, of our not reading the situation correctly, of our being influenced by hidden forces of method (*techne*) or culture (which is carried along by *techne*). As a search for concrete goods, CEC requires that we maintain appreciation for what exceeds our knowing and our doing. CEC techniques in the middle voice, or the mode of *poiesis*, will match the kind of endeavor we are engaged in, bringing into view the goods toward which we aim, which are contextual goods.

CEC, then, is a kind of doing for which rules and procedures are insufficient. Yet general best practices are still appropriate; they come to be embodied and enacted in the ethicist as she continues to rehearse the unifying of practice and theory, with the intention to behold what exceeds her gaze. Jeffrey P. Bishop describes it well:

> When doing clinical ethics, a master practitioner is not just following a set of rules. She enacts, enlivens, indeed embodies the rules such that they are not mere rules applied, but have become actions aimed at goods. It is even odd to refer to them as rules or procedures at all. She knows which rules to follow and which to reject. She knows which guidelines and policies are unnecessary and which guidelines or policies are indeed made ridiculous given the particulars of an encounter. That means that, second, the rules cannot and should not be reduced to a formal code.[12]

So guidelines, rules, policies, procedures, best practices, etc. have a place in the structuring of CEC yet are intentionally sidelined at the moment of responding to an individual crisis. The techniques we use to approach the individual crisis, in particular, *must be flexible* to allow for the doing of CEC.

The weaknesses of his approach notwithstanding, Richard Zaner offers a clear vision of what kind of doing CEC is: a doing that must be intricately tied to the case itself (concrete engagement with particulars), a doing that co-constitutes the ethical meaning of a case (the ethicist is an implicated actor with a particular set of lenses), and a doing that aims toward the goods of healing appropriate to medicine, which imparts a normative structure. Agich praises Zaner's vision for the primacy it gives to the lived practice itself, for which "there is simply no substitute."[13] Starting from an understanding of CEC from within, the doing of clinical ethics becomes a process of encounter and response, rather than a process of technique implementation. We must always remember that our first reaction to a consultation request ought not be to deploy a method but to engage in an interpretive process of uncovering the structures of ethical meaning involved in the case.

Based on CEC as this type of doing, CEC techniques ought to facilitate the asking of three questions within the looping movement between theory and practice:

(1) What is happening here? (seeing reality clearly)
(2) What could happen here? (engaging moral imagination, trying on possibilities)
(3) What ought to happen here? (venturing a normative decision)

These three questions correspond with core features of ethics: *encounter*, *wisdom/discernment* (in virtue ethics, this is called *phronesis*), and *normativity*, respectively. Even while eschewing standardized methods, we can still embrace intentionality about the questions we ask and the goods toward which we aim. We can also still embrace intentionality about the purpose and movement of practical ethics, so that involved persons understand what an ethics consultation is and what they can expect from the consultation. Everyone who consults ethics has a right to know where they are in the process (even or especially though it is not linear), what the ethicist is doing, and why. In our case study, for example, the ethicist described for Dr. Moore the anticipated next steps and clarified the timeline, which is likely to be different in each case, and which consult requesters have a right to know.

Another important element of the doing of clinical ethics, which counterintuitively does not go without saying, is its inherent and exquisitely close connection to the actual practice of medicine. Despite the recent trend to identify CEC as itself a *practice* in the MacIntyrian sense,[14] CEC is not a practice (i.e., a set of activities aimed at internal goods which are realized in the course of trying to achieve standards of excellence in that activity).[15] Rather, CEC is a set of activities aimed at the goods internal to the practice of medicine. Clinical ethicists came on the scene (in the 1960s and 70s) as medical professionals became overwhelmed with the complexity of modern medical technology and found themselves ill-equipped to answer the myriad moral and ethical questions it posed. It may be that medicine has passed the point of return to the days when doctors were the experts in medical ethics, medicine having become so complex that doctors (and other medical practitioners) require the assistance of someone trained in moral theory and in the study of bioethics. We should not see this relationship as an outsourcing of the moral, because there is no medicine without its morality, but rather as a participation between medical professionals and ethicists in a common search (or struggle, or striving) for the good. Medical practice, qua practice, entails working toward human flourishing and is oriented toward Goodness, Truth, and Beauty. While I cannot offer a sustained exploration of medicine qua practice here, I mean only to point out that medicine too (not only CEC, or not only practical ethics) is oriented toward the good and thus can be understood as a kind of worship.[16]

CEC and the Virtue of *Phronesis*

The "kind of doing" I am describing gains additional dimension and depth when seen through the lens of virtue ethics. Aristotelian virtue ethics has seen a resurgence in medicine in the last 30 years, due largely to the work of Edmund Pellegrino and David Thomasma.[17] Pellegrino and Thomasma offer a virtue-based ethics grounded in the nature and ends of medicine, highlighting fidelity to trust, compassion, *phronesis*, justice, fortitude, temperance, integrity, and self-effacement as key virtues for medical practitioners. *Phronesis* (practical wisdom) in particular fills a special role in clinical ethics as the capacity for discernment of moral choice in concrete circumstances. Even before Pellegrino and Thomasma's influential text *The Virtues in Medical Practice*, Albert Jonsen (1991),[18] Stephen Toulmin (1982)[19], and Alasdair MacIntyre (1981, 1988)[20] each tried to develop a *phronesis*-based ethics of medicine. Others have since added to this important body of literature, including many who connect *phronesis* to medical hermeneutics, in the tradition of Hans-Georg Gadamer.[21] Its appeal then and now, in part, is its constructive response to two of the challenges posed to ethics by postmodernism: (1) that we had become too stuck in theory and removed from actual practice, and (2) that normativity could not be agreed upon by everyone in a secular society. Virtue ethics avoids the abstraction trap (challenge 1) unlike other approaches that favor universal, external morality such as principlism, utilitarianism, and deontology. On the other hand, it avoids slipping into relativism or radical particularity (challenge 2) unlike approaches that attend solely to practice. Virtue ethics unifies theory and practice—indeed, one cannot be virtuous without *practicing* the virtues, but one cannot practice the virtues without *knowing* what they require—which we must do in order to save practical ethics. As Thomasma writes, "Virtue theory . . . is positioned between the abstract and universal on the one hand and the pluralistic and relative on the other."[22]

One of the challenges to a contemporary virtue ethics of medicine is that classical Aristotelian virtue ethics relies upon a coherent metaphysical system within which contentful moral norms and virtues can be articulated and defended, something we do not have in medicine today. However, Pellegrino and Thomasma have always acknowledged that virtue ethics cannot stand alone in our time. Instead of searching for metaphysical agreement, however (such as Tristram Engelhardt does in his turn to particular moral communities),[23] they rely upon MacIntyre's concept of the internal morality of practices/professions to help articulate virtuous action in medicine. According to Pellegrino, "everything depends on the moral structure of the professions."[24] It is from within this structure that we can define virtue, even if we disagree about metaphysics, because "the act of profession and the specific phenomenological context within which it is performed entails certain character traits in the person making the profession."[25] In fact, virtue ethics is particularly well-suited to describe the ethical practice of medicine because of its long history of reflection on professional judgement.[26] When coupled with MacIntyre's work on practices, which richly articulates the primacy of a practice's ends (*telos*) apart from metaphysical agreement, a virtue ethics of medicine helps define the contextual goods toward which the medical profession aims, and the type of actions needed to achieve them.

So virtue ethics is an answer to the postmodernism challenge, but still, more must be said about the nature of the medical virtues in order to be helpful in guiding the actions of clinical ethicists. Virtue ethics' particular strength for clinical ethics is its elucidation of the virtue *phronesis*, practical wisdom, which I identify as occurring largely within the second of practical ethics' three movements:

(1) What is happening here? (seeing reality clearly)
   a. Ethical core feature: encounter
(2) What could happen here? (engaging moral imagination, trying on possibilities)
   a. Ethical core feature: wisdom/discernment/*phronesis*
(3) What ought to happen here? (venturing a normative decision)
   a. Ethical core feature: normativity

There is much to learn from virtue theorists about *phronesis* as our field attempts to answer the question "What kind of doing is CEC?"[27] *Phronesis* (the term used by Aristotle) or prudence (for Aquinas) is the virtue that disposes us to seek truth for the sake of action. For Aquinas and in the Catholic church's moral tradition, prudence is the capstone virtue, the link between the moral, intellectual, and supernatural virtues. It means not only intellectually knowing what is good (deliberatively) but being inclined to do it in particular circumstances (dispositionally).

In Aristotelian terms, medicine is a craft (*techne*) which aims at the desired effect of health. Medical ethics, in contrast, is not a craft (and also not a theory), but involves a *praxis* (*phronesis*) of adjudicating the appropriate means to reach the desired effect of health. Medicine's *techne* is always intimately connected to its *phronesis* because what is "healthy" or "good" for each human body/person cannot be known in advance but must be discerned in each particular case. The practically wise person is one who has learned to attend to the good of the whole person in morally ambiguous and medically complex situations, and who is disposed to seek that good. As Glenn McGee writes,

> A clinical ethics based . . . on *phronesis* will emphasize the irascible qualities of a case, its "lived" and human dimensions. Moreover, it will insist that participants in the teaching encounter face the case at some length and confront it not only in terms of familiar principles but also in its clinical dimensions and in terms of its possible outcomes.[28]

Practical ethicists in every field ought to embody *phronesis* and seek to foster its development in the practitioners we advise.

Phronesis is a virtue, not a method.[29] So while deepening our understanding of what this middle stage of ethical reasoning requires of us and what kind of people we ought to be, *phronesis* itself does not guide our stages of action. The suggestions I will offer in the coming sections are consistent with a *phronetic* approach to practical ethics, which reaffirms that ethics must be done in the mode of *poiesis*. We cannot embody *phronesis* using techniques that challenge-forth and guarantee solutions. As Pellegrino and Thomasma remind us, "Prudence does not guarantee certitude. It recognizes the anxiety of choice in complex circumstances. It does enable us to assess the complexities as accurately as possible and to approximate, as closely as the circumstances permit, what would be right and good . . . "[30]

Locally Building and Evaluating Techniques

Local

I do believe there are ways to perform CEC that remain true to the nature of practical ethics, and in the coming chapters, I will describe such techniques. Yet, before I do so, I want to reflect on a few prerequisites. First, because CEC techniques must allow us to encounter non-identically repeated reality, they cannot be standardized across contexts. Instead, CEC techniques should be local: crafted for a specific context by the person who will be using them. In the upcoming Part II, I will describe some elements CEC techniques ought to incorporate. Yet, remember, "quality" ethics is not a matter of uniformity; CEC done well looks different in each context and for each non-identically repeated person. As Agich writes, "Because ethics consultation occurs in circumstances that are unique and dynamic, the consultant must, of course, be open to the circumstances and somewhat flexible in handling the case as it unfolds."[31] That means you, ethicist, must develop for yourself a technique for responding to ethics concerns that incorporates the appropriate elements but nevertheless remains intentionally flexible.

Provisional and Revisable

Next, our locally built techniques are always going to be systematically incomplete, both on an individual level and as a field. Part of the expertise involved in practical ethics is knowing how to fit incomplete approaches to the setting at hand. That does not mean we avoid building them. After all, even while eschewing standardized methodology, the nature of the activity of practical ethics still offers us structure within which to build. Practical ethics requires the use of *techne* of some kind, like all practical endeavors.[32] Just as a qualified ethicist must be well-versed in theories, rules, policies, and procedures, they also must be well-versed in their typical technique in order to be effective. The point is that all of these things—theories, rules, policies, and any "usual procedure" or technique—ought to be in a feedback loop with actual circumstances in their emergence, which may often call for their modification. Techniques for practical ethics must be provisional and revisable.

Evaluable

Ethicists should not flounder in the dark creating ad hoc approaches to consultation requests, but should rather create local techniques informed by practical reason that are revisable and interruptible by the vicissitudes of reality. Such techniques ought to be evaluated, both by ethicists themselves and the wider ethics community, for congruence with a responsible pursuit of the good. I echo Marian Gray Secundy's disquiet with what she calls the "failure of scholars to take risks in unpacking the value-laden assumptions" underlying the techniques we use, are taught to use, or claim to use.[33] If our actions (even those originally non-standardized) become uncritical habits, rules, or traditions invoked unreflectively, and if those actions become routine and accepted by the surrounding medical environment, then we are in danger of losing the critical reflection that makes CEC what it is.[34]

As we found in Chapter 1, humans are essentially technological creatures whose very bodies and existence are co-constituted by interaction with our tools, processes, and habits. The creation and deployment of techniques are powerful actions; techniques shape us, techniques delineate the possible moral outcomes, and techniques help determine our mode of relating to being(s). Techniques are not just neutral tools we can pick up and set back down. They help us see and work with a certain ontological reality, which has profound impacts on the human lifeworld. Through contextually developed, interruptible CEC practices, we can be formed to (however imperfectly) see reality as it is and is becoming, and seek the contextual goods possible in the crises which occasion ethics consultation. How will we know a good technique when we see it? Evaluation must be a continual element of technique development—just not the kind of evaluation used in challenging-forth. Rather, the types of questions which can guide our evaluation of CEC techniques in a liturgical stance might include: "What does this technique reveal or obscure about the nature of being?" "To what am I attuned by this technique, and to what does it blind me?" "Since humans are co-constituted with their technologies/techniques, what kind of person do I become as I relate to this technique?" "How does this technique influence the relationships between me and others (patients, families, co-workers)?" and "How does this technique define and communicate the roles and responsibilities of the clinical ethicist?" We must ethically assess our ethics techniques knowing that our techniques shape both our ethics and ourselves as ethicists; they determine our perception, shape and delimit the moral possibilities, and even help determine the future of practical ethics.

Clinical ethics consultants ought to regularly create space for self-reflection and peer review, not just while they develop their techniques but continuing—

repeated with a difference—as they go about their work. For example, this can be a practice of accountability and self-reflection taking place in peer groups. In my work, I participate in two such groups, one with peers outside of my institution and one with colleagues inside my institution. Importantly, the evaluation of techniques and practices cannot be done in the abstract but must be connected to actual cases and engaged by the person who is developing, using, and revising the techniques in their practical setting. Something personal is at stake for the ethicist in their work as a participatory practice. Part of the purpose of self and peer review is to develop ourselves, in community, into the kinds of people who can hold this work.[35] Frolic and Rubin describe the kinds of accountability that are appropriate for clinical ethicists:

> Just as we offer a response to the classic question of ethics when we are called to offer ethics consultation in specific cases—what is the right/good act and what makes it so?—so too ought we be able to offer a normative defense of our practice—what was the right/good way to approach this case, what makes that so, and how well did we do in upholding that standard? We need to be able to offer an account and a defense to ourselves and to our peers, not only of what we did, but why we did it and why we thought it was the good or right thing. We need to be able to describe: our thinking and underlying rationale; the beliefs, assumptions, and biases that guided our choices; the tradeoffs or compromises we may have consciously or unconsciously been willing to make; and how we might have allowed ourselves to be impacted by the external constraints under which we have been asked to practice.[36]

Professional accountability is still possible without proceduralism and rules; in fact, perhaps even more so:

> Given that the "technical" dimensions of ethics consultation involve moral deliberation ... critical reflection on the question, "Where do I stand in this?" is particularly crucial: What life experiences, commitments, allegiances, insider knowledge, and prior cases might be shaping my analysis of the case? How do my own histories and biases influence how I approach stakeholders, how I comport myself, what I say and when? An ethics consultant, even one who is an outsider to the organization, cannot articulate the "view

from nowhere" and all of us (being human) have particular moral blind spots. Humbly, we must acknowledge the influences on our behaviors and thoughts, and in some cases, we might even need to disclose these influences to others to ensure the integrity of the process.[37]

So while retrospective self and peer review should take place at regular intervals, Frolic and Rubin additionally describe a critical self-reflection that can and should take place *as we engage* in the daily work of consultation, education, and policy review. Our CEC techniques should integrate time to regularly ask ourselves throughout the day or week: Am I being true to my role? Am I doing my best? Is it making a difference?[38] Is love the center and end of my action? Practical ethics is a moving affair; we must be able to move with it, with integrity.[39]

As this Interlude comes to a close, you might be thinking CEC sounds like hard and vague work; I believe it is, and it demands quite a bit of the ethicist. CEC requires that we become certain kinds of people: practically wise, flexible, discerning, humble. In performing our locally built, provisional, revisable, evaluable techniques for discerning the good, we come to embody the qualities needed. As Agich concludes, we can only learn this expertise by doing the work, not by memorizing or learning procedures in advance. His words are instructive for all practical ethicists:

> The knowledge of any doing or practice is properly and primarily expressed in the doings themselves, the actions that make up the practice. Like all practical activities, competence in ethics consultation is fundamentally acquired through experience, through learning and repetition, and not primarily through cognitive or intellectual learning. For novices in ethics consultation, the articulated rules or guidelines can help, but experienced ethics consultants, like experienced practitioners in any field, operate with rules in the background as it were. The rules come to be embodied and habituated in the actions of competent ethics consultants as they do in competent practitioners in any field.[40]

Let us carefully craft techniques in the mode of *poiesis* which enable us, over time, to embody the kind of difficult doing that is CEC. Just how these techniques ought to look is the subject of Part II.

Notes

1. Aristotle, *Nicomachean Ethics*, Book III, Chapter V, Project Gutenburg, https://www.gutenberg.org/cache/epub/8438/pg8438-images.html.
2. These questions are borrowed from Frolic and Rubin, "Critical Self-Reflection as Moral Practice: A Collaborative Meditation on Peer Review in Ethics Consultation," 50.
3. Thompson, "What Is Practical Ethics?"
4. George J. Agich, "What Kind of Doing Is Clinical Ethics?" *Theoretical Medicine and Bioethics* 26, no. 1 (2005): 7–24.
5. Edwin L. Battistella, "What Is the Middle Voice?" in *OUPblog: Oxford University Press's Academic Insights for the Thinking World* (Oxford: Oxford University Press, 2019).
6. Jan Gonda, "Reflections on the Indo-European Medium I," *Lingua* 9 (1961): 55.
7. Ibid.
8. Ibid., 64.
9. For example, Derrida, Heidegger, Eckhart, and Pickstock. For a couple of secondary explorations of this theme, see Neil Taylor, "Derrida's 'Middle Voice': Writing as Difference and the Textual 'Limits' of Our World" (University of Sussex, 1997).; David Lewin, "The Middle Voice in Eckhart and Modern Continental Philosophy," *Medieval Mystical Theology* 20, no. 1 (2011): 28–46.
10. It seems that Derrida was using the middle voice to argue against Cartesian dualisms rather than Kant, but the same applies. Taylor, "Derrida's 'Middle Voice': Writing as *Difference* and the Textual 'Limits' of Our World."
11. Meanings drawn out of Derrida by Taylor: ibid.
12. Jeffrey P. Bishop, "Doing Well or Doing Good in Clinical Ethics Consultation," Finder and Bliton, *Peer Review, Peer Education, and Modeling in the Practice of Clinical Ethics Consultation: The Zadeh Project*, 184. This book is licensed under the terms of the Creative Commons Attribution 4.0 International License (http://creativecommons.org/licenses/by/4.0/). No changes were made.
13. Agich, "What Kind of Doing Is Clinical Ethics?", 15.
14. For some examples of this trend, see Judith Andre, *Bioethics as Practice*, ed. Allan M. Brandt and Larry R. Churchill, Studies in Social Medicine (Chapel Hill, NC: The University of North Carolina Press, 2002), Friedrich, "The Pitfalls of Proceduralism: An Exploration of the Goods Internal to the Practice of Clinical Ethics Consultation"; George J. Agich, "The Question of Method in Ethics

Consultation," *American Journal of Bioethics* 1, no. 4 (2001): 31–41, and "What Kind of Doing Is Clinical Ethics?"

15 Alasdair MacIntyre, *After Virtue* (London: Bristol Classical Press, 1981), 175.

16 Jeffrey P. Bishop, "On the Liturgical Consummation of Any Future Enhancement," *Christian Bioethics: Non-Ecumenical Studies in Medical Morality* 31(2) (2025): 112-120.

17 Edmund D. Pellegrino, *The Philosophy of Medicine Reborn: A Pellegrino Reader* (Notre Dame, IN: University of Notre Dame Pess, 2008); Edmund D. Pellegrino and David C. Thomasma, *The Virtues in Medical Practice* (New York: Oxford University Press, 1993); *The Christian Virtues in Medical Practice* (Washington, DC: Georgetown University Press, 1996).

18 Albert Jonsen, "Of Balloons and Bicycles--or--The Relationship between Ethical Theory and Practical Judgment," *Hastings Center Report* 21(5) (1991): 14-16.

19 Stephen Toulmin, "The Tyranny of Principles," *Hastings Center Report* 11(6) (1982): 31–9.

20 Alasdair MacIntyre, *After Virtue: A Study in Moral Theory* (Notre Dame, IN: University of Notre Dame Press, 1981); Alasdair MacIntyre, *Whose Justice? Which Rationality?* (Notre Dame, IN: University of Notre Dame Press, 1988).

21 Fredrik Svenaeus, "Hermeneutics of Medicine in the Wake of Gadamer," *Theoretical Medicine and Bioethics* 24:5 (2003), 407-31.

22 Ibid.

23 Engelhardt, *The Foundations of Bioethics*.

24 Edmund D. Pellegrino, "Professing Medicine, Virtue Based Ethics, and the Retrieval of Professionalism," in *Working Virtue: Virtue Ethics and Contemporary Moral Problems*, ed. Rebecca L. Walker and Philip J. Ivanhoe (Oxford: Oxford Academic, 2007), 61.

25 Ibid., 62.

26 Joseph Dunne, *Back to the Rough Ground: Practical Judgment and the Lure of Technique* (Notre Dame, IN: University of Notre Dame Pess, 1997).; Mark G. Kuczewski and Ronald M. Polansky, *Bioethics: Ancient Themes in Contemporary Issues* (Cambridge, MA: MIT Press, 2000).; Pellegrino, "Professing Medicine, Virtue Based Ethics, and the Retrieval of Professionalism."

27 For some examples, see Glenn McGee, "Phronesis in Clinical Ethics," *Theoretical Medicine* 17 (1996): 317–28; Sylvia D'souza and Lucas D. Introna, "Recovering Aristotle's Practice-Based Ontology: Practical Wisdom as Embodied Ethical Intuition," *Journal of Business Ethics* 189, no. 2 (2024): 287–300; Jane Kelley Rodeheffer, "Practical Reasoning in Medicine and the Rise of Clinical Ethics," *The Journal of Clinical Ethics* 1, no. 3 (1990): 187–92.

28 McGee, "Phronesis in Clinical Ethics," 326.
29 Pellegrino and Thomasma, *The Virtues in Medical Practice*, 85.
30 Ibid.
31 Agich, "The Question of Method in Ethics Consultation," 35.
32 Some scholars who correctly identify CEC as a special kind of doing that doesn't fit into procedural standards seem to go a little too far in their refusal of processes or techniques. For example, Bishop rightly argues that CEC is a local form of moral enquiry, seeking to enact human goods which are not captured by (procedural) goals. Yet he fails to note that all practices aimed at goods contain disciplines, canons, and guidelines that include *goals* on the way to the achievement of those internal goods. He writes, "in order to be a practice, CEC must pursue goods, not goals." This is true in an ultimate sense, but practices do not preclude the use of techniques for the achievement of goals on the way to goods. For example, a farmer will plant crops (a goal-oriented technique) on the way to the goods associated with the practice of farming. The important part is that the goals, procedures, and techniques do not define or determine when a practice has been done well. Rather, the achievement of goods determines when the practice has been done and done well. Applying this reasoning to clinical ethics, CEC need not be a "floundering about," as Bishop advocates, but should rather be an intentional, good-guided activity in a liturgical stance. I suspect his phrase "floundering about" is actually a proxy for the features of liturgical-stance techniques, including existential humility, interruptibility, encounter, reciprocity, etc. See Bishop, "Doing Well or Doing Good in Clinical Ethics Consultation," in Finder and Bliton, *Peer Review, Peer Education, and Modeling in the Practice of Clinical Ethics Consultation: The Zadeh Project*, 179–92.; and Bishop, Fanning, and Bilton, "Of Goods and Goals and Floundering About: A Dissensus Report on Clinical Ethics Consultation."
33 She is directly discussing hidden and enacted rules of method, such as those George J. Agich calls us to examine. Marian Gray Secundy, "Thinking about Clinical Ethics," *American Journal of Bioethics* 1, no. 4 (2001): 59.
34 This point is made by Agich in "Narrative and Method in Ethics Consultation," in Finder and Bliton, *Peer Review, Peer Education, and Modeling in the Practice of Clinical Ethics Consultation: The Zadeh Project*, 143–4.
35 Frolic and Rubin, "Critical Self-Reflection as Moral Practice: A Collaborative Meditation on Peer Review in Ethics Consultation," 52.
36 Ibid., 60.

37 Ibid., 52.
38 Questions adapted from ibid.
39 Ethics so practiced can become a kind of spiritual practice. Here I am inspired by the work of Simone Kotva, especially in Simone Kotva, *Effort and Grace: On the Spiritual Exercise of Philosophy* (London: Bloomsbury Publishing, 2020).
40 Agich, "Narrative and Method in Ethics Consultation," 142.

Part II

Practical Ethics as Liturgical Activity

5

The Liturgy's Participatory Ontology

It is first through [rituals] that time and space receive a form that makes the experience of the world possible at all. —Ola Sigurdson[1]

An ICU nurse, Maggie, calls the ethicist one afternoon with a new consult request. Her patient Ravi has been intubated for nine days following an anoxic brain injury. While initially the extent of his brain damage was unknown, two days ago it was determined that Ravi had such an extensive injury that he was not expected to recover consciousness. "He is not brain dead, but he is pretty close," she says, "and I don't know why we are still doing all of this to him." Maggie reports the medical team is getting frustrated knowing their efforts are "in vain" and that "no one will set any boundaries with the family, who wants everything done."

The ethicist decides, upon hearing Maggie's reports of moral distress and frustration, to reach out to the attending physician for his perspective and to suggest a team meeting. The attending reiterates the patient's poor prognosis and says attempts at discussing goals of care with the family have resulted in hurt feelings and increasing resistance to any suggestion of moving Ravi to another facility. He is happy to participate in a team meeting.

When they gather, the medical team shares more of their discomfort with the case. The ethicist leads them in a discussion of relevant bioethics concepts, such as medically inappropriate treatment, futile care, surrogate decision-making standards, and moral distress. While the conversation contains moments of disagreement, the team leaves on the same page regarding the source of their frustration: disagreement with Ravi's family about acceptable goals of medical care. They realize they feel uncomfortable not because keeping a patient like Ravi alive is futile (strictly speaking, it isn't), and not because it is causing him to *suffer (he is unlikely to have any conscious experience), and not even because it is using scarce resources (there is no equipment or medication shortage). They feel uncomfortable because they don't believe keeping alive patients who lack the capacity for conscious awareness is an acceptable goal of medicine.*

Next the ethicist convenes a care conference with select members of the medical team and the patient's family, focusing on goals and, more fundamentally, desired goods. The family shares that they maintain hope for his recovery. The medical team shares in frank terms the unlikelihood of recovery. The family then shares tearfully that, at the very least, they are content for him to receive all treatments necessary to maintain his heartbeat. "As long as his heart is beating, to us, it is worth it. And we know he would feel the same." While the ICU team remains in disagreement over whether such an existence is good for Ravi, they see and understand the family's perspective. They explain why it is necessary that Ravi is transferred to a long-term care facility rather than continuing in the ICU, a transfer which the family reluctantly accepts.

Practical ethics interlaces practice and theory, and practical ethics techniques ought to be created, revised, and evaluated locally. But how can we know whether our flexible, locally built and evaluated techniques reveal ontological truth, or just confirm our theoretical assumptions and biases? I believe the only way to approach being(s) while both remaining open to what will surprise us *and* affirming our access to the good and true is to do so liturgically. Another way of saying this is that the only way to encounter being(s) and what is good in/for being(s) is in a stance, or mode of action, that mirrors liturgical practice such as that of the Christian Eucharistic liturgy.

In contrast to our *ersatz* liturgies in CEC, the Christian Eucharistic liturgy teaches us to approach the world as fundamentally mysterious, surprising, and arriving in the mode of gift. In the liturgy, the world discloses itself to us. We are displaced as the center of reality, our gaze is disrupted and transformed; we are shown that things are emergent, and that we are more interconnected and contingent than we could have imagined.[2] We are othered by Christ, who becomes the primary being-as-such.[3] At the same time, we are reassured of our participation in the story of Goodness, Truth, and Beauty, so that we need not escape ourselves to access reality and the good inherent in it. While the activity of practical ethics is not itself worship, it can be done worshipfully: with the humble stance that the liturgy demands of us, "thus drawing everyday life towards a ritual mode."[4] CEC in a liturgical stance has the capacity to interlace practice and theory. We can approach being(s) using a provisional technique, yet be on the lookout for ways our technique won't match the situation. We can both maintain ethical theory yet be confronted and interrupted by the vicissitudes of reality. And we, as ethicists, can be implicated in our encounters with others in such a way that we are changed by them. Liturgical practices are practices of participation which allow for encounter and for the doing of practical ethics.

Like techniques, the liturgy contains rubrics for action: things are done in a certain way in a certain order for a certain purpose. Also like techniques, the liturgy is a structured activity which co-creates with its human participants an ontology of the perceived world. It teaches us truths about the world as we engage with it. In these ways, the liturgy is very much like techniques in the mode of *poiesis*, which are characteristically flexible to context yet aimed toward specific identifiable goods that transcend context. Yet, unlike techniques (in either of Heidegger's modes, *poiesis* or challenging forth), the liturgy is not wielded by its users to achieve their desired result. As we participate in the liturgy's activity, we are formed to see the world in light of an encounter with the risen Christ. In liturgical formation and encounter, we are changed *ourselves*—not *by* ourselves, but by God. Certainly this is a "result" of liturgical action, but the direction of agency and effect is reversed. I will continue to describe liturgical action in the coming pages, cognizant of the fact that the liturgy is technique-like in some respects but is not a technique in many other respects. It is the liturgy's divergence from usual human techniques that will be most instructive for practical ethicists.

Liturgical action is crucial for the betterment of practical ethics because it troubles the power ontologies I have described as operative in standardized CEC methodologies. In fact, the liturgy is the activity *par excellence* for problematizing the entrapment of challenging-forth and its attendant ontologies. Or, in Jeffrey P. Bishop's words, "The Divine Liturgy itself must become the counterpoint of the modern technological liturgics ... Only Divine Liturgy can withstand the logic of modern technics."[5] Again, techniques are processes which co-create with their users ontologies of the perceived world.

They do so by revealing and concealing certain features of the world, or we could say, by ordering perception. This ordering of perception in turn orders our doing. If modern *techne* constrains human doing toward expediency, efficiency, and efficacy, and objectifies subjects as matter standing in reserve, the Eucharistic liturgy is the inbreaking activity which fosters a new vision of ontology, a new ontic.[6] The liturgy is thus a formative praxis that makes real for us a *participatory* ontology, rather than one of power and separation.[7] The liturgy's ordering of perception toward participation can lead us to an ordering of doing toward participation.

Since we are turning back toward ontology, it will be helpful to clarify how this chapter is situated with respect to Chapter 2. I argued in Chapter 2, following Catherine Pickstock, that being(s) consist of non-identical repetition, helping to explain why standardized technique, which looks for identical repetition, misses being(s). While her work is much more systematic and complex than I could afford to explain in that chapter, here I will take a theological angle on ontology that includes (and goes beyond) my basic description of Pickstock's philosophical reology. I will unite philosophical and theological ideas to describe the liturgy's construction/revealing of being(s), taking cues from Klaus Hemmerle, a twentieth-century German bishop of the Roman Catholic Church, who writes, "In the reciprocal relationship between theology and philosophy, there lies, perhaps, even today, a chance for the reconquest of ontology; this would be significant for theology and for philosophy."[8] This focus on ontology is not meant to distract from Christian theological particularities (creation, Incarnation, Crucifixion, Resurrection, the Holy Spirit, ecclesiology, scripture, etc.). Rather, the aim is to reclaim a thoroughly Christian view of the reality of being, taking all of these theological teachings as sources for understanding. A Christian ontology must be centered on Christ and on revelation, rather than dialectical logic; the "Platonist-Christian" ontological synthesis (as Hans Boersma calls it) maintains this focus even as it delves into metaphysical/philosophical realms.[9] This approach is, of course, consistent with the work of Pickstock and other Radical Orthodox theologians.[10]

Throughout the coming pages, I will refer to this Christian ontology as participatory ontology. There are other names that can be used; in Part I, I explained participatory ontology has been called the *analogia entis*. It has been alternatively termed a Trinitarian ontology,[11] a sacramental ontology,[12] or a relational ontology[13] (all for good reasons), but I will use the term participatory ontology for the sake of consistency.[14] Also, as I describe the way being appears to us in the doing of the liturgy, it is important to remember that separating *the ontology revealed by* the liturgy from *the liturgy itself* is somewhat superficial. Its being and its doing, like that of other techniques, are intertwined even if conceptually distinct.

Finally, I must address an obvious concern in any examination of "the" liturgy: namely, that there is no one universal liturgy to turn to. Within the Christian tradition, there are Eucharistic liturgies in the Roman Catholic Church, the various Orthodox traditions, the Anglican Church, and many Protestant denominations. What is more, within each of these groups, there are multiple variations of liturgy, not to mention the changes that have taken place within all of the liturgies over the past millennia and will continue to take place in the future. There is fruitful scholarship that centers around the critique of liturgical variations, but my argument will avoid such critique. For the sake of the present exploration, the fact that the liturgy is multiplicitous and variable across time and space can be considered a reflection of its refusal to become just another standardized and ossified technique. I will incorporate insights from Catholic, Anglican, Orthodox, and Protestant scholars, but when I discuss the liturgy, I will be thinking most clearly about the one I practice, which is the Episcopal Rite. Lines from prayers will be taken from the *Book of Common Prayer*, either Rite I or II as noted.

Liturgical Ontological Revealing

As we begin to explore what is revealed to be true about things (*res*) and being (*ens*) in the Eucharistic liturgy, we will notice that some very strange things happen metaphysically in the liturgy that do not happen in other techniques. In fact, even the taken-for-granted backdrops of time and space are reconfigured. Hans Boersma writes that the liturgy reconfigures *time*; it insists that every temporal event in ordinary time derives its meaning and significance from the Christ event.[15] Time is centered around, interpreted through, and consummated in Christ. In the liturgy, we are simultaneously in the past (the historical events of Christ), the present (this new reconfiguring and reenacting), and the future (the consummation of time in the eschaton). This is especially true in the Eucharist. John Zizioulas writes, "The eucharist is thus the affirmation *par excellence* of history, the sanctification of time."[16] The liturgy also reconfigures *space*; in the Eucharist, the earthly thing, bread, gets taken up into the heavenly body of Christ. In the words of consecration, the thing, *res*, in this time and space comes to participate in eternity and transcendence without losing its integrity as *res*, as bread. In an intensification of the already ongoing participation of *res* in *ens*, in the Eucharist, time and space come to sacramentally participate in eternity such that ordinary bread and wine become "for us" the Body and Blood of Christ.[17] So, a very strange metaphysics is at work indeed.

Partly because of the liturgy's renegotiation of time and space, distinctions and separations between things begin to fall away or to have new meaning. Pickstock terms it a "radicalization of dichotomies such as inside and outside, before and after."[18] We pray that we might be able to pray; we travel towards the pure altar by finding a pure place within ourselves; within and without are ambiguous.[19] The usual dichotomies are radicalized to the point of falling apart, so that not just time and space but even subjects and objects are reconfigured and woven together. "It seems to me," writes Boersma, "that the shape of the cosmic tapestry is one in which earthly signs and heavenly realities are intimately woven together, so much so that we cannot have the former without the latter."[20] In the liturgy's dismantling and retelling of dichotomies, we see that *res* and *ens* are sacramentally connected: the created world points to God as its origin and continual source of being.

This connection or participation of *res* in *ens* was articulated, stammeringly yet firmly, in the thinking and writing of the early Church fathers. As Zizioulas recounts, in the ancient Greek context in which Christianity emerged, the dominant ontology was Platonic, which had an extreme monism at its heart: the being of God and the being of the world formed an unbreakable unity.[21] The church fathers recognized some truth in the Platonic ontological story but insisted that God had freedom with regard to the world. God did not *need* to create, God freely *chose* to create. Because God is utterly free, Platonic monism does not sufficiently explain being.[22] On the other hand, the fathers rejected Gnosticism's dualistic claim that an insurmountable gulf exists between the divine and the earthly realm.[23] Thus, to preserve both divine freedom and participation between God and creation, the church fathers developed an ontology out of their ecclesial experience; or in other words, out of what they were taught about the world by their liturgical and sacramental practice. They developed the "Platonist-Christian" ontological synthesis, which was "perhaps the greatest philosophical achievement of patristic thought"[24] according to Zizioulas. It is this ontological synthesis that is revealed in liturgical action.

The liturgy's participatory ontology has many theological connection points which will be woven throughout this chapter. There is no way to divorce ontology from theology in this paradigm. Theologically, in Thomistic language, we could say "participatory ontology" means that God creates and sustains the world through Christ's emanation from the Father; thus, the created order actively participates in the being of God as exemplified in the Trinity.[25] Participatory ontology ultimately affirms that the observable appearance of creation points to and participates in the eternal mystery of God. It is thus an ontology that secures transcendence while also securing the integrity of the immanent *res*. *Res* cannot be fully comprehended by mere observation and cannot be reduced to measurable dimensions.[26] Just as the sacraments of the church point to the mysterious presence of God in material reality, the being of creation is a sign of the Mystery that is present in and transcends material reality. Therefore, we can call the Christian ontology both sacramental and participatory: like the sacraments, the *res* of our world are not intelligible apart from the Being of God; they participate in a greater reality from which they derive their being and value.[27]

Things Are Mysterious and Cannot Be Mastered (Revelation)

While certainly not exhaustible here, several elements of liturgy rise to the forefront when we begin to look for the liturgy's ontological revealing. For one, things are always arriving in the mode of *gift*. The direction of gift-giving is ambiguous at times, but the origination of giving is always beyond us. For example, in the words of consecration before the Eucharist, the priest says to

God, "Bless and sanctify . . . these thy gifts and creatures of bread and wine; that we, receiving them . . . in remembrance . . . may be partakers of his most blessed Body and Blood (Holy Eucharist, Rite I)."[28] The priest acknowledges *even as he or she is offering them to God* that bread and wine are originally gifts *from* God ("these thy holy gifts which we now offer unto Thee (Holy Eucharist, Rite I)."[29]) And as the priest petitions God for blessing and sanctification of these gifts, there is assurance that God will "show them to be holy gifts for [His] holy people . . . the Body and Blood of [His] Son Jesus Christ (Eucharistic Prayer D, Rite II)."[30] God gives the bread and wine to us, we give them back to God, and God gives them back again as Jesus' own Body and Blood.

Gift-giving is intricately tied to revelation, which is present in every movement of the liturgy. Before the sacrament of the Eucharist is received, the congregation hears the word of God, the scripture passages for the day, which are understood to be divine revelation. Revelation is the original gift which makes the approach to God possible—as in the liturgical progression, so also metaphysically. Revelation comes in various forms in the liturgy, not just as scripture, and all of it leads to God's fullest revelation, that of Godself in the person of Christ. In the liturgical progression, the Old Testament passage is heard first, then the Psalm, then the New Testament, and finally the Gospel. The liturgical movement leads from the words of ancient revelation in scripture and tradition to The Word, Jesus Christ. (Notice that this highest revelation, the person of Christ, is a revealing that stands in contrast to the revealing/concealing characteristic of *techne*.) Revelation's coming to us from beyond us, like the gifts of bread and wine which God and the people mutually offer to one another in the Eucharist, teaches that only God is the original source of truth and knowledge.

A proper humility is thus required. In order to receive the word from God, we have to prepare ourselves. In the Collect for Purity, the Gloria, and the Collect of the Day, spoken or sung before the scripture readings, the people give glory to God and request mercy to receive revelation from God. Lines of glory and petition are repeated-with-a-difference several times at the opening of the Rite, which suggests that the approach to God must be re-begun and circled back around.[31] There is no straight line to the altar, for approach requires the worshipper to divest themselves again and again of sin and presumption. "The prelude to arriving at an altar is not simply a temporo-spatial journey, but also a preparation of the self, a putting-on or putting-off to render oneself fit for, or partially protected from the divine presence . . . "[32] writes Pickstock. This process reminds the congregation that the approach to God is not a simple one and is not completed by our own power. Rather, God comes to us and speaks, and God's word is ever new and ever beyond us. The liturgy teaches us that things are mysterious and cannot be mastered, that truth and understanding come from above.

The liturgy's use of paradoxical language constantly reminds us of the mysterious nature of the world, which has been given to us from outside ourselves. Pickstock writes,

> [The liturgy's] language is in several ways impossible, for liturgy is at once a gift *from* God and a sacrifice *to* God, or reciprocal exchange which shatters all ordinary positions of agency and reception, especially as these have been conceived in the West since Scotus. Moreover liturgical expression is made impossible by the breach which occurred at the fall. This breach is the site of an apparent *aporia* for it renders the human subject incapable of doxology and yet . . . the human subject is constituted (or fully central to itself) only in the dispossessing act of praise. However, the *aporia* is resolved in the person of Christ, whose resurrection ensures that our difficult liturgy is not hopeless and enables us to rejoin the angelic liturgy taking place in an ambiguous and shifting space beyond our own.[33]

Thus liturgy is "an expectant work, the hope that there might be a liturgy."[34] We have no power or control to wield. The world is gifted and in many ways unknowable in its fullness. In liturgical action, the mystery of Christ's incarnation leads us further into the mystery of the world. God became man; our Other came and dwelt among us, interrupting, calling, communicating, revealing.[35] As Hemmerle writes,

> . . . that which is other than everything and different from everything nevertheless becomes something within everything's horizon, becomes something concrete amongst what is concrete. Religion is grounded in the transcendent's making an incursion into immanence without giving up its claim to be transcendent.[36]

In Jesus Christ, we encounter a God who encounters us.

The mysterious nature of the world, having received its being from the Being of God, requires a decentering of the self of the worshipper. In liturgical action, unlike the other techniques we have examined, the one who performs it is not the one who guarantees its completion. In Pickstock's words,

> [The] one who calls upon God is one to whom God in turn speaks, thereby situating the unidentified worshiping "I" with which the Rite opens, not only within a shifting place, but also within a relational place, in an I-Thou relationship with the ultimate Thou . . . The calling "I" does not occupy a prior or more primitive subject-position, because God alone makes the cry both possible and audible.[37]

The action of the liturgy thus represents a reversal of the typical way techniques function. The worshipper does not move through the steps of liturgical action in order to arrive at the desired conclusion or problem resolution. In fact, the worshipper does not wield the liturgy as a technique at all. The worshipper only gradually comes to occupy a subject position as God allows. Insofar as it could be considered a technique, it is one wielded by God, who alone can ensure the worshipper's arrival at the end of the liturgy. The primary "technique user" turns out not to be the worshipper at all, nor even the priest. Worshippers and priest are swept up into the ritual action through which God shows them reality (again: revelation, as opposed to revealing/concealing). Techniques co-construct with their users an ontology of the perceived world; in liturgical action, God breaks into this construction with revelation from outside us.

A disruption of the usual direction of agency leads to new relational possibilities. The relational reversal and reconstitution between the worshipper and God happening within the liturgy is what Pickstock calls the "liturgical I-Thou relationship." This relationship "involves a ceaseless struggle for the worshipper, for whom the secular assumptions of empirical priority and instrumentality . . . inimical to voice, gift, and redemptive sacrifice, perpetually threaten to suspend the ontologically necessary liturgical dispossession of the 'I.'"[38] The worshipper must be decentered and dispossessed in order for the liturgy to move forward, requiring a constant putting off of old ways of relating, and an embrace of new relational structures. As Pickstock notes, this is both an ontological necessity and a constant struggle, for all of us are steeped in opposing metaphysical assumptions.

Things Are Relational (Trinity)

As the liturgy moves us toward revelation, gift, mystery, and the reversal of agency, it is teaching us about the nature of being(s). In the liturgy, we are shown that God is the fountain of all being, and God is relational, for God is the One in Three Persons. Not only do all *res* participate in *ens*, but *ens* is fundamentally relational itself. Existence is always already relating. Zizioulas writes that the church fathers' understanding of the being of God (directly connected to their ecclesiology and liturgical practice) rests on the following two affirmations: (1) There is no being without communion, and (2) Communion which does not come from a *concrete and free person* leading to other *concrete and free persons* is not of God.[39] "The person cannot exist without communion, but every form of communion which denies or suppresses the person, is inadmissible."[40] The primacy of communion of persons guided the patristic theologians (the church fathers) in their doctrine of the being of God (and thus creation) as *relation*. Communion thus becomes an ontological concept: nothing is conceivable in itself without communion, not even God.[41]

As we saw in Chapter 4, much of modern philosophy remains stuck on the dilemma posed by Kant. Having accepted that the "inside" of a person is fundamentally unconnected from the "outside" of a person, philosophers center their ontological reflections around an epistemic problem. But the question of how to connect the "inside" with the "outside" is misguided from the perspective of Christian participatory ontology. As Rowan Williams says, human existence is always inseparable from intelligent reaction to what is not ourselves. "Our identity is always already shaped by *response*."[42] Being(s) are never entirely self-contained because they are constantly in the process of moving out from self-identity into relation, or rather "realizing identity in a relatedness that is never absent."[43] Things are constantly relating to other things and therefore always in *motion* out from themselves. The liturgy reinforces this relational movement when, after their confession of sin and the priest's assurance of forgiveness, the congregation moves to greet one another with a sign of peace. Fundamental peace with God allows peace with neighbor.

In a participatory ontology, a *res* can only be understood in its action, its motion. A thing's motion constitutes and communicates its being and varies according to context. This sounds, of course, like what Pickstock describes as the non-identical repetition of being(s). Pickstock writes of the movement of being(s) in their non-identical repetition through space and time as a movement like a serpent, waving, curling, folding, a partial return initiating each novel forward motion.[44] Williams says it this way: "What *is* is in motion, and not only in motion but in a motion that includes otherness in its own action and definition."[45] According to Hemmerle, only Trinitarian language can capture this understanding of being. Things are in motion toward an other; being arrives to an other in the mode of self-gift (rather than the philosophical "given").[46] Because of the Trinity, says Zizioulas, "not only communion, but also *freedom*, the free person, constitutes true being. True being comes only from . . . the person who loves freely."[47] Thus we have arrived at the ontological foundation, according to the Christian liturgy: free self-giving, which is to say, love.

Love and Self-Giving Are the Foundations of Things (Creation, Incarnation, Trinity)

The theological justification of a participatory ontology is God's gift of Godself—in creation, in the Incarnation, Passion, and Pentecost, and ultimately in the perichoresis (the "moving around" or "rotating") of the Trinity.[48] I will discuss all of these facets together, in an attempt not to overly systematize them. As we are reminded through participation in the liturgy, in creation God gives permission to God's other to be itself. "At your command all things came to be: the vast expanse of interstellar space, galaxies, suns, the planets in their courses, and this fragile earth, our island home. *By your will they were created and have their being* (Eucharistic Prayer C, Rite II)."[49] And in Eucharistic Prayer D, "Fountain of life and source of all goodness, you made all things and fill them with your blessing; you created them to rejoice in the splendor of your radiance (Rite II)."[50] God speaks and *res* come into existence, participating in *ens* but never exhausting it. God's created other is granted the freedom to be its own particular manifestation of being, not just according to its form but unique within its form. This is so important that Maximus the Confessor uses two different terms to refer to these aspects of being: *logos* and *tropos*—*logos* being akin to a form, and *tropos* the fluid way in which a thing manifests its form.[51] The *logos* defines *what* a thing is, and the *tropos* defines *how* a thing is, which is unique to it.[52] While ontologies of power run into problems of equivocation, as described in Chapter 2, in a participatory ontology "the unequivocality of a form in itself corresponds to its equivocal reference beyond itself."[53] In the act of creation, the Trinitarian God allows difference to come into being, while maintaining relationship with it. But of course, this allowing of difference is not a singular phenomenon in creation, but flows from the nature of God as Trinitarian incorporation of difference. "Difference in God is the source of the difference of the creation from God,"[54] as Andrew Davison says. By virtue of its creation by a Trinitarian God, a *res* is both distinctly itself and a member of the plurality of not-itself.

But God's hospitality to the other does not stop with creation. In the Incarnation—then again in the Passion, Resurrection, and Pentecost—God gives Godself over to God's other.[55] "In the fullness of time you sent your only Son, born of a woman, to fulfill your Law, to open for us the way of freedom and peace (Eucharistic Prayer C, Rite II),"[56] we hear in the Eucharistic Prayer. Or, "you, in your mercy, sent Jesus Christ, your only and eternal Son, to share our human nature, to live and die as one of us, to reconcile us to you, the God and Father of all. He stretched out his arms upon the cross and offered himself, in obedience to your will, a perfect sacrifice for the whole world (Rite II)."[57] In becoming human, Christ demonstrated "an 'ecstatic' relation with the Father, a radically self-emptied and other-directed love."[58] Rowan Williams writes,

> In both creation and incarnation, God has elected to live within the created order without ceasing to be what God eternally is. What God brings about in the finite is a movement of "desire," *eros*—that is, a movement beyond what the intellect can master and a growth in love.[59]

Williams explains that the union of divine and human in Christ is thus the "pivot of a metaphysic" in which integration and reconciliation can be realized in the world.⁶⁰ The borders between self-contained individuals are permeable, and our connections with others run deeper than we imagine.⁶¹ Even the suffering of Christ in the Passion is a "playing out [of] the dependence and joyful self-offering of the Son to the Father, true for all eternity, but under the conditions of a sinful world."⁶²

God's own very existence as Trinity is love and self-giving, an internal unity of three Persons. The three Persons of the Trinity relate to each other in a way that can be described as co-inherence, reciprocation, intercommunion, mutual indwelling, and interpenetration, all meanings that have been historically captured in the Greek term perichoresis.⁶³ But to separate God's doing—God's self-giving in creation, the Incarnation, and the giving of the Holy Spirit—from God's being as self-giver is superficial. The *analogia entis*, participatory ontology, is thus grounded in the self-giving of the Trinity to all creation. Here lies the twofold mystery that God is both *self-giving in Godself* and *self-giving toward what is not God*. God's self-giving is the pure beginning of being. "*Analogia entis* means Being's reciprocal into-each-other and out-of-each-other. This for-each-other unconceals itself as the meaning of this Being,"⁶⁴ writes Hemmerle. All being(s) are enfolded in the mystery of love, the mystery of free self-giving:

> The analogy of Being becomes, also, an analogy of the Trinity. Everything fulfils itself and brings that which is its ownmost to perfection by entering into its relatedness, into its being-beyond itself, into its self-having as self-giving, into its character as to and for each other.⁶⁵

Thus, as we learn in the liturgy, the Trinity is not a logical abstraction, but a statement of the fundamental experience of being. "All Being experiences a radical turning if God is the threefold, and, as the threefold, has His history in our history,"⁶⁶ writes Hemmerle. In fact, the Christian liturgy reconfigures the persons gathered such that they can experience full participation without loss of self, which mirrors the mystery of the Trinity.⁶⁷ Suddenly, the ontological foundation of the world is love and relation, transforming epistemology as well. As we are taken into the life of the Trinity through the liturgy and its mediated participation in Christ, a new relationality is opened between us, as *res* in the world. Hemmerle thus has the basis to claim that being-in-Christ opens a *Trinitarian relationship* between created beings, a relationship that allows for participation without loss of self.[68] The participation of creatures in one another is a reflection of the divine participation of the persons of the Trinity.[69] Maximus the Confessor agrees, writing that because God creates and sustains all things, God "providentially binds the intelligible and the sensible things *to one another* and to himself."[70] Further,

> [God] makes the things that have been set apart from one another by nature to be the things that have converged with one another by the one power of their relationship with him as their beginning. And it is by this power that all things are led to an identity of movement and existence that is indistinguishable and without confusion.[71]

While differing from each other in nature and motion, all *res* remain united with all other *res*, according to their one relationship with the Creator. This one relationship "nullifies and covers over" all individual relationships, not by abolishing them, but by surpassing and outshining them, allowing the totality to come into view rather than the parts.[72] As the Trinity exists as substantial unity of three Persons without confusion, God creates in the world a "oneness by nature without confusion around the substances of the things that are, alleviating and making identical that which is different around them by the reference to and oneness with himself . . . "[73] Maximus continues by insisting that here the natural differences and distinctions between *res* do not cause alienation between them; power and separation need not mark relationships between things. Rather, "[God] encloses all things in himself . . . just as a center defines the lines that originate straight from it."[74] In this peaceful relatedness which is love, Maximus says being(s) are safe from the danger of changing into non-being, which is separation from God.[75] In other words, here again free self-giving love is the ontological foundation.

For one more example, Bonaventure writes that revealed love is the ontological core of creation.[76] Drawing on Bonaventure, Hemmerle posits that what becomes central, if love is core to being, is the movement of *relatio* from self to other.[77] Therefore, "Only one thing remains: active participation in that movement which *agape* itself is. This movement is the rhythm of Being; it is the rhythm of giving that gives itself."[78] Here the problem of phenomenology is resolved; the empirico-transcendental doublet is no longer necessary because the epistemic enterprise is already in the process of life itself. When we go along with the process of life itself, which is love and self-giving, "it is revealed what is going on, who is going on, and whence and whither the process is going."[79] To the one who enters into this movement of self-giving, of love, is permitted an *encounter with being*, which subsequently invites a response, a decision.[80] Thus, we have made our way from metaphysics to ethics (if they can be so disentangled).

What Participatory Ontology Does Not Mean: Rejecting Pantheism

Inherent in this ontology is a warning. As C. S. Lewis explains,

> The books or the music in which we thought the beauty was located will betray us if we trust to them; it was not *in* them, it only came *through* them. ... These things ... are good images of what we really desire; but if they are mistaken for the thing itself, they turn into dumb idols. ... For they are not the thing itself; they are only the scent of a flower we have not found, the echo of a tune we have not heard, news from a country we have never yet visited.[81]

As I have argued elsewhere, Christians have consistently pushed back against a doctrine of participation that allows for idolatry or pantheism.[82] Creation is not an ultimate reality in itself, then, but a sign of (yet more than a sign, an analogy of) the ultimate reality of God. Material creation's existence is derived from a source external to it, and thus always points beyond itself to what is ultimately important, which is heavenly reality.

Zizioulas takes pains to emphasize that participatory ontology is not radical monism; it does not threaten the unique identities of individual *res*. He says, "It is only in relationship that identity appears as having an ontological significance, and if any relationship did not imply such an ontologically meaningful identity, then it would be no relationship."[83] While creation actively participates in God, creation is not God; God is beyond all things. John of Damascus writes, "He is the being of all things that are, the life of the living, the reason of the rational, and the intelligence of intelligent beings . . . [and yet he] surpasses intelligence, reason, life, and essence."[84] Since God is the source of all being(s), God cannot be another *res* among *res*. The Fourth Lateran Council of 1215 affirmed, "For between creator and creature there can be noted no similarity so great that a greater dissimilarity cannot be seen between them."[85]

Andrew Davison offers another way to understand this: "God is *not* the material cause: creation is not made *out of* God. Neither, on the other hand, is matter some rogue element, unmade by God, unrelated to him, and outside his control. God is not the material cause but God is the cause of matter."[86] Thus it has been said that while creation participates in the being of God, God *communes* with creation.[87] God and the world have a relationship of ontological otherness bridged by love.[88]

Practical Ethics with a Participatory Ontology

In this chapter, we have explored the liturgy's ontological revealing, with the thesis that the liturgy is the activity *par excellence* for problematizing challenging-forth. The liturgy reveals to us an ontology in which the world is mysterious, surprising, gifted, and not under our control—and yet we have access to the good and true already by nature of our being. We are displaced as the center of reality, our own power is disrupted and transformed; yet grace beyond ourselves secures us. A proper humility is required, enabling new ways of relating. If *res* participate in *ens*, a participation characterized by the nature of *ens* as free self-giving love, then an encounter between beings is possible. This encounter is an analogy, an *analogia*, for the Trinitarian mutual indwelling of God.

Still, what does liturgical action and its ontological revealing offer us as practical ethicists? What does it teach us about our work, about the techniques we should use in CEC? How does this ordering of perception order our doing? In the next chapter, I will arrive at a vision of CEC as a moral activity in the "middle voice," terminology previously reclaimed by Radical Orthodox theologians Milbank and Pickstock, and described in the Interlude. To be faithful to a participatory ontology as ethicists means that we must practice new ways of relating. The good and true is to be found in the encounter with the persons before us, not in safely arriving at the completion of a technique. Our knowledge and control cannot lead us all the way. Being is mysterious and surprising; we must have eyes to see it, while not losing sight of the theories and thought structures of which our expertise partly consists.

The case study at the beginning of this chapter is an example: the ethicist did not enter the team meeting or the care conference with pre-formed recommendations or theories to apply. She did bring, however, knowledge of concepts which helped to delineate the themes at hand (or found to not be at hand), including futile care, medically inappropriate treatment, surrogate decision-making standards, and moral distress. Only in conversation with the medical team could she know which ethical themes were causing their concern and begging to be explored. From a procedural standpoint, she did not have a predetermined step-by-step process to resolve the conflict. However, she was able to follow her typical consult structure:

(1) What is happening here? (seeing reality clearly)
(2) What could happen here? (engaging moral imagination, trying on possibilities)
(3) What ought to happen here? (venturing a normative decision)

in a flexible way that embraced a humble stance of participation with others. The process allowed for the expression of familial love to hold normative weight while also empowering the ICU team to set an appropriate boundary, i.e., transfer to long-term care.

To correct for our over-reliance on procedures in clinical ethics, we must embrace a lot more mystery, an understanding of being as a gift from outside ourselves. A search for the good of being(s) in concrete situations can no longer be considered straightforward, a matter of implementing the right techniques and procedures to secure quality. Yet, there are things to be said about the type of techniques we should use, and the elements or features appropriate for techniques in ethics. Formed by a liturgical stance, we must be interruptible and we must allow for genuine disagreement and diversity. Our stance cannot be one of mastery, but of humility: we will often find ourselves in the face of situations and people we do not fully grasp. But this humility in the face of mystery, this beholding of reality, is not a radical skepticism or relativism. It is not an abandonment of normativity or a collapse into empiricism. It is a constant relinquishing of power and control in order to participate more fully in the good which is already in being itself.

Notes

1 Ola Sigurdson, *Heavenly Bodies: Incarnation, the Gaze, and Embodiment in Christian Theology*, trans. Carl Olsen (Grand Rapids, MI: William B. Eerdmans Publishing Company, 2016), 415.
2 Pickstock, *After Writing: On the Liturgical Consummation of Philosophy*.
3 For more, see Simmons and Benson, *The New Phenomenology*; Thomson, *Heidegger on Ontotheology*.
4 Pickstock, *After Writing: On the Liturgical Consummation of Philosophy*, 174.
5 Jeffrey P. Bishop, "Technics and Liturgics," *Christian Bioethics: Non-ecumenical Studies in Medical Morality.* 26, no. 1 (2020), 27–8.
6 The relationship between ontology and ontic is complex in Heidegger and in other Continental philosophers. I use the word "ontic" here to denote an ontology that concerns particular, individual beings rather than categories about being. While Heidegger writes about the ontic as an isolation of a being to the particular, losing its significance within the whole of being, in light of Pickstock's work I see ontic as an idea worthy of reconsideration. Perhaps we need not view attention to the concrete as an abandonment of ontology, but as a corrective.
7 See Hans Boersma, *Eucharistic Participation: The Reconfiguration of Time and Space* (Vancouver, BC: Regent College Publishing, 2021).
8 Klaus Hemmerle, *Theses Towards a Trinitarian Ontology*, trans. Stephen Churchyard (Brooklyn, NY: Angelico Press, 2020), 14.
9 Hans Boersma, *Heavenly Participation: The Weaving of a Sacramental Tapestry* (Grand Rapids, MI: William B. Eerdmans Publishing Company, 2011), 20–21. John Zizioulas agrees that the patristics' ontology was a fusion of platonic and Christian theological ideas; see John D. Zizioulas, *Being as Communion*, ed. Kallistos of Diokleia Christos Yannaras, Costa Carras, Contemporary Greek Theologians (Crestwood, NY: St. Vladimir's Seminary Press, 1985). Pickstock's work also reflects this synthesis.

10 For an overview of Radical Orthodoxy, see John Milbank, Catherine Pickstock, and Graham Ward, eds, *Radical Orthodoxy: A New Theology* (London: Routledge, 1999).
11 Hemmerle, *Theses Towards a Trinitarian Ontology*.
12 Boersma, *Heavenly Participation: The Weaving of a Sacramental Tapestry*.
13 Christos Yannaras, *Relational Ontology*, trans. Norman Russell (Brookline, MA: Holy Cross Orthodox Press, 2011).
14 There may be nuanced differences between the ontologies described by these different names. My analysis will avoid such nuance and focus instead on a level of agreement that can be found generally across Christian traditions.
15 Boersma, *Eucharistic Participation: The Reconfiguration of Time and Space*.
16 Zizioulas, *Being as Communion*, 22.
17 Space does not permit a robust consideration of these themes, but for an excellent exploration of the liturgy's space and time, see Pickstock, *After Writing: On the Liturgical Consummation of Philosophy*, especially Chapters 4 and 5.
18 Ibid., 220.
19 Ibid., 186.
20 Boersma, *Heavenly Participation: The Weaving of a Sacramental Tapestry*, 24.
21 Zizioulas, *Being as Communion*, 16; See also Andrew Davison, *Participation in God: A Study in Christian Doctrine and Metaphysics* (New York: Cambridge University Press, 2019).
22 Zizioulas, *Being as Communion*.
23 Ibid.
24 Ibid.
25 Thomas Aquinas, "Summa Theologiae," (2017; reprint, Online Edition), First Part, Question 45.
26 Boersma, *Heavenly Participation: The Weaving of a Sacramental Tapestry*, 21.
27 Ibid., 24.
28 Episcopal Church, *The Book of Common Prayer and Administration of the Sacraments and Other Rites and Ceremonies of the Church* (New York: Church Publishing Incorporated, 1789), 335.
29 Ibid.
30 Ibid., 375.
31 Pickstock, *After Writing: On the Liturgical Consummation of Philosophy*, 169–219.
32 Ibid., 186.
33 Ibid., 176–7.
34 Ibid., 186.

35 Hemmerle, *Theses Towards a Trinitarian Ontology*, 24.
36 Ibid., 24–5.
37 Pickstock, *After Writing: On the Liturgical Consummation of Philosophy*, 196.
38 Ibid., 197–8.
39 Zizioulas, *Being as Communion*, 18.
40 Ibid.
41 Ibid., 17.
42 The word "response" is often used in relation to revelation: God reveals, we respond, and are saved. But Williams is saying response is not only an agential turning to God confined to the "moment" of salvation; rather, response is always already operative in our very being. Rowan Williams, "Foreword," in Hemmerle, *Theses Towards a Trinitarian Ontology*, 2.
43 Williams, "Foreword," ibid., 2.
44 Pickstock, *Repetition and Identity*, 21–40.
45 Williams, "Foreword," in Hemmerle, *Theses Towards a Trinitarian Ontology*, 2.
46 Williams, "Foreword," ibid., 3.
47 Zizioulas, *Being as Communion*, 18.
48 Hemmerle, *Theses Towards a Trinitarian Ontology*, 51.
49 Episcopal Church, *The Book of Common Prayer and Administration of the Sacraments and Other Rites and Ceremonies of the Church*, 370, italics indicate congregation response.
50 Ibid., 373.
51 Maximus also extends the *logos-tropos* pairing to Christ, explaining how Christ participates in the Father and in humanity. See Davison, *Participation in God: A Study in Christian Doctrine and Metaphysics*, 211–12.
52 Ibid., 211–12.
53 Hemmerle, *Theses Towards a Trinitarian Ontology*, 47.
54 Davison, *Participation in God: A Study in Christian Doctrine and Metaphysics*, 53.
55 Hemmerle, *Theses Towards a Trinitarian Ontology*, 60.
56 Episcopal Church, *The Book a Common Prayer and Administration of the Sacraments and Other Rites and Ceremonies of the Church*, 370.
57 Ibid., 362.
58 Rowan Williams, *Christ the Heart of Creation* (London: Bloomsbury Continuum, 2018), 107.
59 Ibid.
60 Ibid., 121.

61 Ibid.
62 Davison, *Participation in God: A Study in Christian Doctrine and Metaphysics*, 214.
63 These terms are offered by Andrew Davison. Ibid., 56–7.
64 Hemmerle, *Theses Towards a Trinitarian Ontology*, 46.
65 Ibid., 52.
66 Ibid., 32.
67 For more on this point, see chapter 9 of Sigurdson, *Heavenly Bodies: Incarnation, the Gaze, and Embodiment in Christian Theology*.
68 Hemmerle, *Theses Towards a Trinitarian Ontology*, 55.
69 Davison, *Participation in God: A Study in Christian Doctrine and Metaphysics*, 52.
70 Saint Maximus the Confessor, *On the Ecclesiastical Mystagogy*, ed. John Behr, trans. Jonathan J. Armstrong, Popular Patristics Series (Yonkers, NY: St. Vladimir's Seminary Press, 2019), 51, italics added. In this work, Maximus presents an allegorical-eschatological reading of the liturgy which is not entirely relevant here but deserving of future scholarship.
71 Ibid., 51–2.
72 Ibid., 52.
73 Ibid., 55.
74 Ibid., 54.
75 Ibid.
76 Hemmerle, *Theses Towards a Trinitarian Ontology*, 33. See Saint Bonaventure, *Holiness of Life* (London: Forgotten Books, 2018; repr., Classic); *The Works of Bonaventure: Cardinal Seraphic Doctor and Saint: Volume I. Mystical Opuscula*, trans. Jose de Vinck (Quick Time Press, 2020).
77 Hemmerle, *Theses Towards a Trinitarian Ontology*, 35
78 Ibid.
79 Ibid., 37.
80 Ibid., 51.
81 C. S. Lewis, *The Weight of Glory* (New York: Harper Collins, 2001), 30–1.
82 Jordan Mason, "Transhumanism, Motion, and Human Perfection," *Christian Bioethics* 28, no. 3 (2022): 185–96.
83 Zizioulas, *Being as Communion*, 88.
84 *On the Orthodox Faith*, I.14, in John of Damascus, *Writings*, trans. Frederic H. Chase (Washington, DC: Catholic University of America Press, 1958).
85 Canon 2, in *Decrees of the Ecumenical Councils: From Nicaea I to Vatican II*, vol. 1 (Washington, DC: Georgetown University Press, 1990), 232.

86 Davison, *Participation in God: A Study in Christian Doctrine and Metaphysics*, 43.
87 Zizioulas, *Being as Communion*, 94.
88 Ibid., 90–1.

6

Practices of Participation, Not Power: Clinical Ethics Consultation Techniques in a Liturgical Stance

For Christian wisdom does not consist in applying rules, nor in confronting what happens with the lessons of a manual, but in making our existence as disengaged, as ductile as possible, so that it tends to be nothing but an Aeolian harp on which the Spirit can improvise, according to the needs of the moment and the exigencies of such an encounter. —Jean-Louis Chretien[1]

"I need to stop the surgery, right? Just give me the word and I'll stop it—I'm not concerned about that. I just can't believe no one else sees this is a problem." The surgeon, Dr. Omar, is exasperated. His sixteen-year-old patient Alexa is scheduled to receive a surgery in two hours, a surgery that she does not want but which was strongly recommended by her oncologist. Dr. Omar goes on to explain to the ethicist that Alexa's mother consented to the surgery, but everyone knows the cancer is so advanced it is unlikely to offer much benefit. And besides, Dr. Omar insisted, Alexa seemed old enough to make her own decisions, even if slightly under the legal age.

The ethicist asks Dr. Omar for more clinical context. He explains that Alexa has been receiving cancer treatment for about a year, but the treatment has been unsuccessful, and as the cancer has spread, her oncologist has recommended more and more surgeries. Previously, Alexa has been agreeable, but this time is different. She looks tired and frail. She asks to go home and to stop fighting, a request her mother quickly silences.

The ethicist affirms Dr. Omar's concerns and tells him she needs to call the oncologist to understand more. There is not enough time to fully engage with

Alexa and her mother in person as she would usually do, but the ethicist promises to get back to Dr. Omar with a recommendation within an hour. She reviews the chart and contacts the oncologist but gets no response. She begins to take notes and jot down various ethical considerations based on other similar situations, such as decision-making for mature minors, "assent" in pediatrics, and medically non-beneficial treatment. Some of these considerations seem relevant in this case, but there is not enough time to draw out their implications or to engage in a moral imagination process.

The ethicist gathers her thoughts and crafts a chart note, describing the potentially relevant ethical considerations, but highlighting her inability to provide a normative opinion on the case as a whole. She therefore offers a recommendation to postpone the surgery until additional conversations can take place. Before signing and posting the note, she calls Dr. Omar to relay the information and recommend that he postpone the surgery. He is unsurprised and relieved, and asks that the ethicist follow up with the case the next day.

The liturgy offers us a new ontic, which undermines the false ontological assumptions operative in standardized CEC techniques. In this chapter, I will explore CEC techniques as liturgical practices of participation, rather than practices of power. We will see how techniques with a liturgical quality (in what I am calling a liturgical stance) allow practice and theory to be mutually referencing and mutually revising. While other CEC approaches privilege one or the other, or allow one to exercise authority over the other, concrete practical concerns and limitations *and* theoretical normative ethics knowledge should remain in tension and in a mutual process of adjustment in each case. Collapsing neither into the empirical/descriptive nor into the exertion of normative control, a liturgical stance invites us into new ways of relating: both of relating practice and theory, and of relating the ethicist and other persons. And interestingly, these two types of relations turn out to be connected. A liturgical stance offers us a way to conceive of ethical action in the middle voice, where actors are both active in and passive to their doing. In short, liturgical practices are practices of participation which allow for encounter, and thus have the capacity to transform CEC.

A main goal here is to offer concrete suggestions for features that I believe should be at the heart of CEC techniques in a liturgical stance. Yet I have argued that, given the non-identically repeated nature of reality and the type of activity CEC is, developing and using CEC techniques in a liturgical stance must be the work of each individual ethicist in their own context. Thus, I will not offer a standardizable method or identify steps for CEC in a liturgical stance. To do so would place my suggestions right back in line with other standardized techniques that challenge forth. Rather, I will suggest a few core features that will be common to all varied CEC techniques in a liturgical stance. The features I discuss ought not to be considered exhaustive; they are merely a starting point for further discussion and development among clinical ethicists and within various practical contexts. A participatory ontological foundation will shape our doing, but it will not dictate in advance what actions should be taken.

Because the features I highlight are not direct guidance for the technical "doing" of CEC (intentionally so), we will be forced to evaluate CEC techniques and practices in ways other than procedural correctness. Still, as described in the Interlude, ethicists should both be able to evaluate their own practices on a local level and be held accountable to the wider profession. While professional sources often evaluate techniques based on the values of challenging-forth—things like efficacy, efficiency, repeatability, and reliability—our questions must be different. As I explained in the Interlude, instead of asking questions like "how effective and efficient is this method at finding a solution to the ethical problem?" we should ask questions like, "What does this technique reveal or obscure about the nature of being?" and "To what am I attuned by this technique, and how does it blind me?" A refusal to standardize techniques will not mean ethicists are left to their own devices. Counterintuitively, it will offer us an opportunity to *more deeply* investigate and more accurately perceive how our techniques are shaping our work and ourselves. I invite ethicists to engage these ideas in an ongoing collaborative conversation as they develop CEC techniques.

Some Features of a Liturgical Stance

Interruptibility: Keeping Moral Space and Time Open

As Margaret Walker's famous metaphor of the "ethicist as architect of moral space" suggests, our techniques structure space; they also structure time.² In Chapters 3 and 4, I briefly explored the ways our prominent CEC techniques structure time and space: ways that narrow our attention for the sake of agreement and/or efficient resolution. The liturgy, in sharp contrast, reconfigures time and space, centering them around the person of Christ. It reveals that things are not always as they seem, and that approaches to truth are not linear. Techniques in a liturgical stance will structure time and space in such a way that our bodies and attention are drawn to spaces where the other confronts us.³ CEC techniques in a liturgical stance will reject the usual linear, logical steps that structure other CEC methods. Instead, they will remain committed to interruptibility, which keeps techniques from becoming ossified and rigid, and reflects the understanding that people, situations, and solutions will always exceed our ability to know or grasp them. Interruptibility is a way of keeping moral space and time open, helping us to see more clearly what is, might be, and ought to be as we engage consultations.

Like in the liturgy, CEC techniques should structure time in a non-linear fashion, such that approaches to the good and true are repeated-with-a-difference throughout. Elements of the ethical process should be re-begun and circled back around, so that we strike the proper stance of openness to what we do not expect. Unlike techniques in which "information-gathering" is only one initial step, CEC techniques in a liturgical stance will weave asking, listening, and eliciting the stories of those involved into the entire process. Non-identical repetition is not a mere conceptual category, but an ontic truth that may reveal itself in the course of a consultation if the participants have prepared themselves to receive it by so structuring their activity. In contrast to methods which aim directly toward resolution, those in a liturgical stance will be open to inefficient, slow, and repeating parts of the process if they serve ethical inquiry and are best suited to the particular persons gathered.

Techniques in a liturgical stance will open space for encounter in logistical ways as well as moral ways. Logistically, they will open space by choosing thoughtfully whom to include in the process, where to gather for meetings, how to interact with medical professionals, etc., based on the particulars of the situation at hand. Our techniques should also bias us toward bodily presence with the suffering patient, structuring our attention around the non-identically repeated person on whose behalf the medical team is laboring. Yet, as we see in this chapter's case study, even such a bias must be interruptible due to the constraints and contingencies of time and medical realities. We must have a working idea of which elements of the process will be necessary in order to complete the process and which are not: in the case study, the ethicist was not able to provide normative recommendations on the case as a whole due to her time constraints, so she did not venture to make them; however, she felt confident in recommending that they postpone the surgery to allow the necessary time for seeing reality clearly and for moral imagination.

Techniques in a liturgical stance will open moral space by keeping a wide lens of possibilities. Holding open moral space means drawing on our moral and ethical expertise to situate the emerging contextual crisis or concern within the larger collection of knowledge our training has afforded us. We need not do away with theoretical knowledge, structures, or patterns of thought in order to open moral space; in fact, they are necessary in order to do the job well. However, we must access those crucial resources without sidelining other forms of knowing, and while maintaining openness to revising our theories in light of the present crisis. Knowing that solutions will not come directly from theoretical structures frees us to be able to consult them while also attending to the emerging situation, ready to revise our understanding of either when we are shown to be wrong.

Encounter: Attuning to the Mysterious and Surprising

Within such "open" time and space, an encounter with reality becomes possible. By now, it should be clear that the encounter is a necessary condition of CEC and that standardized techniques can and often do preclude it. It should also be clear that even some non-standardized techniques, such as Zaner's phenomenological method, do not facilitate encounter, at least not as properly defined. How can a liturgical stance enable an encounter with being(s)? In part, it can do so by allowing our preconceptions to be frustrated, allowing us to be surprised by what we did not expect. Being is mysterious and surprising; we must be open to the arrival of an encounter. We know from the liturgy that things arrive as gifts from God, originating beyond us. To correct for our over-reliance on procedures in clinical ethics, we must embrace mystery, an understanding of being as a gift from outside ourselves. The good and true is to be found in the encounter with the persons before us, in the moment of surprise, not in safely arriving at the completion of a technique. Our knowledge and control cannot lead us all the way. Even to reflect academically on this feature of techniques in a liturgical stance is to do it a disservice. George Agich reminds us of the limitations of theory in this area:

> Reflecting on clinical ethics is thus a reflection in the midst of the things themselves, namely, the active engagement in the clinical ethics enterprise itself. There is simply no substitute.... The only grounding that exists for this doing is thus to be located in the particular circumstances of the individual case.[4]

Ethics techniques (when built and assessed locally, and when embodying liturgical features) can attune us to the mysterious and surprising by bringing us back to engagement with people and reality as they are, rather than requiring us to define them according to preexisting categories that are recognizable and workable (i.e., this is a moral distress case, a futility case, a questionable capacity case). Techniques must incorporate the time for and intention of a reciprocal encounter, in which our gaze as objective observers of supposedly uniform reality is interrupted. They can do this, for example, by incorporating and valuing more time spent beholding the patient (even if the patient is not or cannot be an "active participant" in the consult), conversing with peripheral members of the clinical team, and more time spent in clinical spaces without an agenda. Whereas standardized methods encourage users to focus their attention on information and perspectives that confirm their working hypothesis of the ethical question, techniques in a liturgical stance will encourage users to pay attention to surprising and contradictory information about what may be really going on. This has the effect of freeing ethicists from their perpetual "active voice" activity, where they are the heroes of the consult, encouraging them to instead engage with consults in the middle voice. Allowing for divergent perspectives, sometimes routing us off course, sometimes changing our minds, techniques in a liturgical stance will foster in us the ability to hold multiple truths at once, breaking the tyranny of one-directional moral technique.

Reciprocity and Communication: Mutual Participation in the Good

CEC, like all manifestations of practical ethics, is defined by the circumstances actually encountered. Yet CEC requires the ethicist to actively involve their own humanity in their engagement with those circumstances. We must participate in the circumstances of the other, not as removed expert, but as fellow human being. Here, the importance of the middle voice comes more fully into view. As Rebecca Dresser says, "Without a good understanding of what it is like to be overwhelmed by the experience of illness—one's own or that of a loved one—how can the doctor or ethicist appreciate the human situation the doctor must address?"[5] Recognizing the interconnected and participatory nature of being as revealed in liturgical action, ethics professionals must bring their own life experiences to bear on cases, allowing for reciprocity, mutual understanding, empathy, and vulnerability. Agich writes, "Doing clinical ethics becomes less a matter of deploying specific techniques for pre-given ethical problems than an *existential and ethical encounter with the sick* and their need for care."[6] In bringing *ourselves* to consults, we can acknowledge the ways we are affected as we affect others: the truth of middle voice activity. Of course, there is a difference between empathy and projection; like those in helping professions such as therapists and social workers, ethicists must be reflective about the ways they might be bringing too much personal feeling into a consultation and sidelining the experiences of those they are trying to help.

Yet we are active participants in the unfolding narrative of each ethics case, not merely observers or experts applying knowledge.[7] Active participation is a crucial difference between *beholding being* and *deploying a gaze* upon it. Being is fundamentally relational; there is no being without communion. From the moment we respond to a consultation request, we are shaping the case as it proceeds, and it is important that we be aware of our impact (and the impact on us), both for reviewing and revising our approach as needed and for properly documenting the consult.[8] The fact that ethicists impact (and are impacted by) the case on which they are consulting is not to be considered a detraction. Taking responsibility for our participation is part of the process. Agich suggests, "Ethics consultation is best understood as a reflective practice and . . . the ethics consultant should be a reflective practitioner who is intentionally aware of and responsible for the actions and communications routinely undertaken in the course of an ethics consultation."[9] Ethicists join and participate in a search for the good that has already begun by the time we enter the scene. Others have begun the search, and to those others we must also be accountable for our actions and impact.

In this chapter's case study, the ethicist may have been moved by Dr. Omar's emotion and hence inclined to offer him the support he needed to postpone the surgery. Being moved to support and elevate a medical professional's moral agency is a beautiful part of clinical ethics consultation, not a hindrance. Yet it is something that the ethicist ought to be aware is influencing her process and her reasoning, especially if she is only able to hear from one participant in the case.

Humility and Reflection: Dealing with Our Error

A liturgical stance requires ethicists to be in the sometimes uncomfortable position that the worshipper occupies in the liturgy: decentered and divested of power and control. While authority and leadership are appropriately given to clinical ethicists, who are looked to in times of distress, our stance must be one of humility and awareness of our own limitations. As we recognize and acknowledge our limited understanding of each particular situation, especially with regard to the patient and family who are usually strangers, we must be ready to revise our ethical theories as well as our processes and techniques as new features emerge. The ethicist's own marginalization is important in CEC because it offers an opportunity to escape the logic of modern *techne*. As Moyse warns, techno-ontology's moral machinery "instrumentalizes knowing for the purposes of doing, and bureaucratizes both the control and the management of persons surveyed by the panoptic gaze and corresponding judgement of technique." Stepping out of the illusion of control breaks the techno-ontological gaze.[10]

Yet there are costs associated with humility and reflection. Just as it is difficult for ethicists to acknowledge the problematic nature of our standardized techniques, it is difficult for us to engage with the uncertainty and chaos of medical-moral crises without the firm footing of procedural certainty. As discussed in the Preface, standardized techniques offer many benefits for individual consultants and the field at large. They offer increased professional accountability and status. They demonstrate the value of ethics to medical institutions. They help us train new ethicists more efficiently. Perhaps most saliently, they help to distance consultants from the demanding nature of our work and from personal responsibility or distress in difficult cases.

Yet ethics has always been demanding personal work. Dietrich Bonhoeffer offered exceptional clarity on the provisional nature of ethical knowledge and the deep personal cost that comes with the faithful pursuit of concrete goods in the context of ethically troubling situations.[11] He writes, "A man with a *conscience* fights a lonely battle against the overwhelming forces of inescapable situations which demand decisions."[12] Seeking to salve the conscience brings only uncertainty and timidity, rather than the boldness and critical distance that aid a normative decision. Ethicists are called to stand in the breach, so to speak, not to hide behind procedure for the sake of their conscience. It comes with uncertainty, which requires a prayerful humility and a willingness to notice when we fail to uncover the good. In fact, the nature of the work ensures that we will not always uncover the good, either because of our own failings or the tragedy of a broken world.[13]

To admit our fallibility starts with letting go of techno-ontological procedural control, but extends to interpersonal accountability for times when we fall short. When we do err, we must be ready to confess and seek reconciliation.[14] Opportunities for this type of interaction are sorely lacking in health care, and it may be that CEC techniques ought to include liturgical processes for confession or lamentation.[15] Techniques in a liturgical stance do not challenge-forth solutions and do not ensure satisfactory solutions can or will always be reached. At the center of techniques aiming to solve moral problems without looking beyond themselves is pride. Our modern Western manifestation of idolatrous pride may look different than in cultures where idols take the form of physical objects or talismans, but it is no less sinful. Techniques may have become our idols. The presumption that the "right" technique will secure ethical outcomes is our distinct manifestation of an age-old quest for power.[16] Our techniques are *ersatz* liturgies when they take on this presumption, when the "ceremonial aspect" of CEC (as Agich calls it) remains *ceremonial* rather than *liturgical,* indicating a harnessing and wielding of institutional power.[17]

Summary

I have argued that standardized techniques threaten the integrity of practical ethics. I began in Part I with a philosophical critique of technique. In Chapter 1, I used Heidegger's philosophy of *techne* to argue that techniques are a kind of *techne*, which means that they are modes of revealing which humans enlist to conceptually construct the world around them.[18] This construction or revealing also implies a concealing, since some aspects of reality must fade into the background as others come front and center. I differentiated between techniques that bring-forth and are thus able to facilitate an encounter between persons, and techniques that challenge-forth solutions to problems and are thus prone to overlooking the very persons we aim to help. In Chapter 2, I argued that standardized ethics techniques challenge-forth, foreclosing on practical ethics by operating within ontological frameworks that are at odds with reality and cannot facilitate an encounter. I relied upon Catherine Pickstock's work to describe being as non-identical repetition, participating in forms yet always appearing anew. In Chapter 3, I showed how four popular CEC techniques, the Four Boxes Method, Clinical Pragmatism, Bioethics Mediation, and the VA's CASES Method, all demonstrate challenging-forth rather than bringing-forth, and thus constitute *ersatz* liturgies. They only reveal the aspects of being they are set up to reveal; they are like self-fulfilling prophecies or echo chambers reinforcing ontologies of *identical* rather than non-identical repetition.

Yet merely rejecting standardization is not enough to solve the problems of technique in practical ethics. In Chapter 4, I examined Richard Zaner's phenomenological method and concluded that phenomenology is still in need of metaphysical reorientation. I reiterated that the facilitation of encounter is a necessary condition for practical ethics, and an encounter is only possible within a participatory framework.

In Part II, I turned to theology to understand the type of action that can facilitate encounter. I identified the Christian Eucharistic liturgy as the model for action that allows us to encounter being(s). The liturgy troubles the ontologies of standardized technique, revealing a radically different ontology of participation rather than power. A few features of a participatory ontology are: (1) things are mysterious and cannot be mastered, (2) things are relational, and (3) love and self-giving are the foundations of things. In this chapter, I described what ethical techniques in a liturgical stance (reflecting and revealing for us a participatory ontology) might look like. While I resisted offering any directives, I suggested that ethicists build techniques that incorporate interruptibility, encounter, reciprocity and communication, and humility and reflection. These elements embody the liturgy's stance toward being(s) and help us approach non-identically repeated reality while at the same time holding onto our expertise/knowledge.

Notes

1 Used with permission of Fordham University Press, from Jean-Louis Chretien, *Under the Gaze of the Bible* (New York: Fordham University Press, 2014). Permission conveyed through Copyright Clearance Center, Inc. Chretien, *Under the Gaze of the Bible*, ed. John D. Caputo, trans. John Marson Dunaway, Perspectives in Continental Philosophy (New York: Fordham University Press, 2015), 42.
2 Walker, "Keeping Moral Space Open."
3 Maximus talks about the liturgy's structuring of space as a blueprint for being confronted. See Saint Maximus the Confessor, *On the Ecclesiastical Mystagogy*; Walker, "Keeping Moral Space Open."
4 Agich, "What Kind of Doing Is Clinical Ethics?" 15.
5 Quoted in Finder and Bliton, *Peer Review, Peer Education, and Modeling in the Practice of Clinical Ethics Consultation: The Zadeh Project*, 14. This book is licensed under the terms of the Creative Commons Attribution 4.0 International License (http://creativecommons.org/licenses/by/4.0/). No changes were made.
6 Agich, "What Kind of Doing Is Clinical Ethics?" 16, italics added.
7 Ibid., 10.
8 This was originally noted and explored in 1999 by Zaner and colleagues: Richard M. Zaner, ed. *Performance, Talk, Reflection: What Is Going on in Clinical Ethics*

Consultation? (Dordrecht: Kluwer, 1999); Mark J. Bliton and Stuart G. Finder, "Strange but Not Stranger: The Peculiar Visage of Philosophy in Clinical Ethics Consultation," *Human Studies* 22 (1999): 69–97.

9   Agich, "Narrative and Method in Ethics Consultation," 141.

10 For an excellent critique of CEC methodology which uses the techno-ontological gaze to privilege the secular over the religious, see Ashley Moyse, "Malek's Programmatic Secularism? A Dissent," *Christian Bioethics* 28, no. 2 (2022): 99–108.

11 Bonhoeffer, *Ethics*.

12 Ibid., 69, italics original.

13 Bonhoeffer writes that the only way for the ethicist to exercise wisdom is to be seized by the love and command of God and thus freed from agonizing indecision. "Not fettered by principles, but bound by love for God, he has been set free from the problems and conflicts of ethical decision. They no longer oppress him. He belongs simply and solely to God and to the will of God. It is precisely because he looks only to God, without any sidelong glance at the world, that he is able to look at the reality of the world freely and without prejudice." Ibid., 70.

14 I envision this process mirroring the sacrament of confession, which I previously argued should guide medical error disclosure as well: Jordan Mason, "Confessional Approach to Disclosure of Medical Error," *Christian Bioethics* 27, no. 2 (2021): 203–22.

15 Objections are often raised that confession of error by medical professionals (which would presumably include clinical ethicists) would increase hospital and professional liability and erode public trust. However, this has not been demonstrated to be true; in fact, there is evidence to the contrary. See ibid.

16 See Brian Brock, *Christian Ethics in a Technological Age*, (Grand Rapids, MI: William B. Eerdmans Publishing Company, 2010), 375–6.

17 Agich, "Narrative and Method in Ethics Consultation," 143.

18 I am careful not to use terminology that indicates humans have complete agency over the choice, utilization, or deployment of *techne*, yet even the terminology I am using here falls short. *Techne* and human being are so intertwined that it is not quite true to say we *enlist* it for specific purposes. Rather, as we use it, *techne* helps co-determine our purposes.

Postlude

An ASBH Case in a Liturgical Stance

But what kind of things one ought to choose instead of what, it is not easy to settle, for there are many differences in particular instances. —Aristotle[1]

The liturgy teaches us that we are interdependent, that our identities are communally created, and that we find ourselves most clearly in moments of self-giving love. We live in the middle voice. These ontological truths should shape our doing in CEC—the goods toward which we aim, the processes we use to get there, and the questions we ask ourselves along the way. The possibilities for CEC in a liturgical stance are wider and harder to envision than those of standardized CEC. While the preparation, the education, the experience level, and the standards of knowledge and analytic ability may be the same for ethicists operating in each paradigm, a liturgical stance is a fundamentally different mode of engagement with ethics. Rather than entering into each consult with a prepackaged form or procedure, a liturgical stance requires one to be spiritually prepared and attuned to the moment. Great jazz artists are classically trained, yet show up on stage ready to improvise in response to their fellow musicians. Those who participate in liturgy do so according to their tradition's rubrics, only to realize after many years that they can participate without consciously referring to the rubrics, the written pages. Likewise, great clinical ethicists are well-versed in the literature, arguments, analyses, and theories that comprise academic bioethics, yet answer a consult call ready to improvise in response to the patient, family, and medical team in each unique situation and context. Abstract, theoretical knowledge is vital yet propaedeutic for the activity of practical ethics. To close, I offer this Postlude: a case-based reflection on the implications of my work for a clinical ethics consultation.

In 2017, ASBH issued a case-based study guide called "Addressing Patient-Centered Ethical Issues in Health Care."[2] The study guide was created to supplement previously published educational material for those learning or teaching how to perform ethics consultation in healthcare settings. It contains twelve case studies, each corresponding to certain competency targets in ASBH literature. The cases include self-assessment questions for the learner, accompanied by learning objectives and strategies. As the cases unfold, further questions and learning objectives are provided, as well as an answer key. Here, I will take Case 1 from the study guide and demonstrate how an ethicist approaching the consult in a liturgical stance may proceed and how their actions may be different from the ASBH's ideal ethicist. To reiterate, CEC in a liturgical stance will look different for every ethicist in each situation and institutional context; this case study is merely a musing on liturgical action in CEC, not a directive or prescription.

Case 1. Decision-Making Capacity[3]

Ethics Consultation Request

Dr. Gibson, a consultation-liaison psychiatrist, requests an ethics consultation, asking whether or how a "functional patient can refuse blood products even if they are really needed." The psychiatrist also asks whether the ethics consultant can assist in elucidating and addressing the patient's concerns.

The Case

Charlotte is a 29-year-old woman with a history of post-traumatic stress disorder, depression, Marfan syndrome (a connective tissue disorder), a left-thigh infection, and chronic anemia. She is admitted to the hospital with a low hemoglobin of 5. Her chronic anemia is due to gastrointestinal bleeding from nonsteroidal anti-inflammatory drug (NSAID) use, and administration of blood products is indicated. She refuses a blood transfusion and wants to leave, against medical advice. Her reason for refusing the blood products is that she "feels like someone is invading her body" whenever she receives blood products. She had received one unit of blood products one week ago and felt "completely grossed out." The psychiatrist, Dr. Gibson, is asked to assess the patient's decision-making capacity, or ability to consent to a particular treatment. (Decision-making capacity is specific to the treatment decision at hand and thus is context based.)

Charlotte is willing to discuss her treatment and her refusal of blood products with Dr. Gibson. She states that she was "raped by her neighbor" and cannot endure blood transfusion because it reminds her of this rape, which occurred 10 years ago. Her mother, who is present in the room, says that Charlotte was a student at a top college on an equestrian scholarship when she was raped. Since then, she has experienced "deep depression," suicidal thoughts, nightmares, avoidance, and irritability—although those are currently in remission or well-controlled. Charlotte has been on an antidepressant and a low-dose antipsychotic at bedtime and has been participating in individual therapy with a psychologist for a year.[4]

At this point, the case narrative pauses and the guide asks four questions of the ethicist, each having to do with the bioethical concept of decision-making capacity. Knowledge of key concepts like decision-making capacity (both as a concept and its use in clinical practice) is crucial for clinical ethicists, and yet knowledge of concepts only gets us partway to knowing what is, might be, and ought to be happening in this case. An ethicist operating in a liturgical stance will know and integrate the concept of capacity, but capacity questions will not take a primary place in her initiation of the consult. But the ethicist has not yet been consulted, so we will proceed.

Continuation of the Case

Dr. Gibson asks Charlotte what she understands about her situation. Charlotte says she knows she has really low hemoglobin and that she may collapse, have a heart attack or stroke, or potentially die if it is not corrected. She says her doctors have explained to her that administration of oral iron has failed and that intravenous iron may take weeks to improve her hemoglobin; she also knows that blood transfusion would much more quickly restore her hemoglobin. Charlotte also talks about many other things and is easily sidetracked. Each time, Dr. Gibson tried to redirect charlotte to talk about blood products. A few times, she conflates receiving blood products with surgery, which Dr. Gibson finds concerning. Charlotte has never had surgery, and does not need it now. When he asks her why she continues to talk about surgery, Charlotte says, "Well, receiving blood is like having surgery."

Dr. Gibson determines that Charlotte lacks the capacity to consent to or refuse the blood transfusion on the basis of his assessment of "her reasoning."

He believes that Charlotte is unable to distinguish blood products from semen or receiving blood products from being raped. He is concerned about the "psychotic underpinnings" of her beliefs and finds "her narrative disjointed." Sometimes she says she was "raped 10 years ago by a neighbor and other times she says she was raped 4 years ago by her cousin." He is also concerned that she continued to talk about "refusing surgery," even after he corrected her and explained that receiving blood products is different from having surgery. In his chart note Dr. Gibson writes, "Although Charlotte is very knowledgeable about hemoglobin and what refusing blood transfusion would entail," she could not "appreciate how receiving a blood transfusion is not the same thing as being raped."

Dr. Gibson believes that Charlotte lacks capacity to consent to (or refuse) the provision of blood products. However, he also thinks she is "otherwise functional and communicative." Dr. Gibson does not know "whether or not to honor her refusal of blood products." After all, Charlotte's mother, her legal surrogate, would provide consent for her receiving blood, and the products are medically indicated, but it would be practically and clinically difficult to provide blood products over Charlotte's objections. To do so would require restraints or sedatives to protect her and the healthcare providers, which he believes "is pretty invasive" for "someone so communicative and fairly coherent." At this point, he calls for an ethics consultation, asking whether or how a "functional patient can refuse blood products even if they are really needed." Dr. Gibson also asks whether the ethics consultant can assist in elucidating and addressing the patient's concerns.[5]

By the time the ethicist arrives on the scene, she is aware that the psychiatrist has already begun a search for the good of this patient. In fact, Charlotte has a larger circle around her who have been searching and working toward her good since her rape, including at least her mother and her psychologist. The ethicist knows that her work will be a joining, a participating, a guiding, rather than a handing down of answers regarding who should decide. Realizing that formulas for capacity evaluations (i.e., standards for what counts as appropriate "reasoning," etc.) have already affected the way Dr. Gibson has formulated the ethics consultation question, the ethicist attends to the case without labeling it a capacity case from the beginning. In any case, she will refuse to limit her engagement to the simple answering of an abstract ethics question but will instead attempt to understand the situation from within as fully as possible.

Recognizing the complexity of trauma and mental health, the ethicist may turn her attention away from identifying "the ethics question" at all in this case, turning instead to an encounter with the patient. The ethicist notes the capacity determination and the legal/ethical standards for decision-making but places them to one side as she engages with the deeper question "what is really going on?" To answer this question, she will need to speak with the patient directly and will attempt to do so multiple times: repetitions with a difference. She will not look to narrow down information like Clinical Pragmatism's corkscrew but will embrace the fact that human beings (especially those who have experienced trauma) process, integrate, and share information and values in ways that are complex and even contradictory. This is reflective of life itself. A disjointed narrative should not deter the ethicist from taking the patient's accounts seriously and entering into the patient's experience in order to elicit further the feelings and motivations behind her wishes.

Based on her previous experience in this particular hospital, the clinical ethicist will have developed a technique she usually relies on to move through consultations. The general flow and reasoning behind her technique will have been communicated to her colleagues, and perhaps Dr. Gibson is already aware that she will start by encountering the patient, and then others involved in the patient's care. He might know that she next goes back to her office and writes down the patient's narrative and the impressions she gathered in person, highlighting any areas where additional information is needed; possibly another perspective should be elicited, or additional ethical research is warranted. The ethicist will circle back as often as needed to these sources as gaps in her understanding emerge. Maybe Dr. Gibson often sees the ethicist return to the patient and bedside practitioners and subsequently widen her sphere of information gathering to include those who are not present near the bedside (consulting physicians, social workers, outpatient support, etc.). He knows that she will soon begin to integrate all of the information and impressions she receives and brainstorm how to apply theoretical ethical resources to this particular case, including concepts like decision-making capacity. She may next ask a small team of colleagues on the ethics committee to review her developing case narrative, which will eventually be abbreviated and turned into a chart note when the consult is over. This will create opportunities for peer evaluation of the process as it is unfolding, as well as evaluation of the ethicist's emerging ethical recommendations.

Perhaps in this case, when the ethicist begins by meeting the patient, the interaction proceeds as follows:

> The ethics consultant meets with Charlotte and explains that the purpose of her interview is to try to "learn more about [Charlotte's] concerns about the blood products" and "whether the team can attend to those concerns." Charlotte is agreeable to talking with the ethics consultant and has an open and conversational demeanor. However, because of concern about having Charlotte recount her story yet again to a difference healthcare professional, the ethics consultant asks Charlotte whether telling her story would cause negative or traumatic feelings for her. Charlotte is willing to tell her story and does so with little hesitation.
>
> Charlotte tells a narrative similar to the one she provided to Dr. Gibson. She discusses her rape experience openly and candidly. The ethics consultant asks Charlotte what happened the last time she received blood products. Charlotte says she was "alone" and "scared," and "no one explained what was going into me" or "why I needed to have it right then." Recognizing a potential modifiable barrier that the healthcare professionals could address, the ethics consultant asks whether Charlotte might respond differently if someone were there and if details about the transfusion were explained. Charlotte is unsure and says she needs time to think about this.[6]

At this point, the ethicist begins to think Dr. Gibson's capacity assessment was incorrect and that Charlotte does indeed have capacity. It becomes clear that Charlotte equated the needlessly confusing experience of receiving her last blood transfusion with her rape experience (both were accompanied by fear of severe bodily harm, invasiveness, and extreme lack of control), but not the blood itself. All of the contextual features of the case are integrated into the ethicist's exploration of "what is happening here?" (seeing reality clearly).

*What are the stages of your CEC technique, and how would you have begun this particular consult? Take a moment to write down your process of encountering patients and/or clinicians in moral crisis:*_____

Next the ethicist moves into the moral imagination phase: "what could happen here?" She asks the medical team whether it is medically feasible to wait a number of days before administering the blood transfusion, and they agree to a maximum of 3 days' delay. The ethicist continues her reflective writing process in collaboration with her colleagues, who think she is right to delay the blood transfusion while exploring options with Charlotte. She meets with Charlotte again the next day with a few ideas: would she feel comfortable trying a blood transfusion if the entire process were explained a day in advance, with the ethicist present to help clarify any confusion? Would she feel comfortable if her mother and/or another friend or family member accompanied her? Would she like to choose the time of day? The ethicist offers Charlotte any element of control and choice that is feasible.

In ASBH's case narrative, Charlotte agrees to try one unit of blood as long as her friend Madelyn can be present to hold her hand, and someone explains what is going on. The psychiatrist reassesses Charlotte's capacity and finds that "she may have capacity." Charlotte continues to be willing to receive blood products, which she needs regularly for a few months. The last phase of the consult—normative recommendations: "what ought to happen here?"—has answered itself as the possibilities have taken shape and the patient has led the way. The ethicist is thus spared the decision of whether or not forced treatment was defensible, but perhaps she was prepared with preliminary answers to those questions based on what she had seen so far in this case. In different circumstances, the case could have been complicated by a number of factors: continued refusal by Charlotte, an urgent medical need for the transfusion without time to get Charlotte's approval, continued insistence from the psychiatrist that Charlotte lacked capacity, input from other family members, or disagreements over surrogate decision-making, etc. Each of these factors would have interrupted the ethicist's smooth operation of her usual technique. She would need to speak to additional parties, integrate more information, change her theory about what was really going on, and revisit parts of the process. Importantly, she would need to research and/or recall more and different legal and ethical norms around each eventuality (e.g., under what conditions is it justifiable to force treatment over objection? Is there a legal hierarchy for determining the decision maker? Are there hospital policies governing dispute resolution? How does urgency/emergency change consent requirements?). None of these eventualities would cause concern about the process because interruption would be understood to be a normal part of ethics technique. The "what ought to happen here?" phase of the consult would be a more full-throated normative venture if the case had become complicated by such features. Each case needs a different level of emphasis on each part of the ethics process, but the good of the patient is always the guide.

*What are the middle and ending stages of your CEC technique? Take a moment to write down your process for moral imagining and developing normative recommendations:*_____

_____
_____
_____
_____

As the ethicist reviews her work on the case, perhaps in a monthly peer group, she reflects on the aspects of reality that were revealed and concealed by her approach. Because she knows CEC is an activity done in the middle voice, she recognizes what kind of ethicist she is becoming as she engages in her particular process: is she coming to over-rely on the opinion of the medical team rather than encountering the patient herself? Is she hurrying through any parts of the process to save time? Is she neglecting family members that seem "difficult"? Is she hesitant to offer a recommendation that would make a certain physician uncomfortable? She is held accountable by her peers for her normative recommendations. Do they comport with widely held ethical standards, and if not, why? Can she defend her decisions in a transparent way? And finally, she remembers the patients and families with whom she interacted. Was she open to being corrected, when her theories failed, by those patients who revealed in their lives and bodies some truth she did not yet know? How did love, as the ontological core of reality, motivate her work and change her? Did she deploy a preformed gaze upon the patient, or did she allow herself to behold the patient in their uniqueness? The questions are as varied and endless as the situations in which we find ourselves, here in the strange world of medicine. They are as varied and endless as the people who arrive in our hospitals, each non-identically repeated, and each reflecting the goodness that is at the heart of being itself.

*How do you evaluate your CEC technique? Take a moment to write down your processes for self and peer review:*_____

_____
_____
_____
_____

"By definition [efficiency] must reduce experience to computation, particularity to abstraction, and mystery to a small comprehensibility. . . . And yet love obstinately answers that no loved one is standardized. A body, love insists, is neither a spirit nor a machine; it is not a picture, a diagram, a chart, a graph, an anatomy; it is not an explanation; it is not a law. It is precisely and uniquely what it is. It belongs to the world of love, which is a world of living creatures, natural orders and cycles, many small, fragile lights in the dark."—Wendell Berry[7]

Notes

1 Aristotle, *Nicomachean Ethics*, Book III, Chapter I, Project Gutenberg, https://www.gutenberg.org/cache/epub/8438/pg8438-images.html.
2 American Society for Bioethics and the Humanities, *Addressing Patient-Centered Ethical Issues in Health Care: A Case-Based Study Guide* (Chicago, IL: ASBH, 2017).
3 From American Society for Bioethics and Humanities, *Addressing Patient-Centered Ethical Issues in Health Care*. Copyright © 2017 American Society for Bioethics and Humanities. Reprinted with permission.
4 American Society for Bioethics and the Humanities, *Addressing Patient-Centered Ethical Issues in Health Care*, 7.

5 Ibid., 8.
6 Ibid., 9.
7 Wendell Berry, excerpt from "Health Is Membership" from The Art of the Commonplace: The Agrarian Essays. Copyright © 1994, 2002 by Wendell Berry. Reprinted with the permission of the Permissions Company, LLC on behalf of Counterpoint Press, counterpointpress.com.

Bibliography

"Accreditation Manual for Hospitals." Edited by Joint Commission on Accreditation of Health Care Organizations. Oakbrook Terrace, 1992.

Agamben, Giorgio. *Opus Dei: An Archaeology of Duty*. Stanford, CA: Stanford University Press, 2013.

Agich, George J. "The Question of Method in Ethics Consultation." *American Journal of Bioethics* 1, no. 4 (2001): 31–41.

Agich, George J. "What Kind of Doing Is Clinical Ethics?" *Theoretical Medicine and Bioethics* 26, no. 1 (2005): 7–24.

Agich, George J. "Why Quality Is Addressed So Rarely in Clinical Ethics Consultation." *Cambridge Quarterly of Healthcare Ethics* 18, no. 4 (October 2009): 339–46.

American Society for Bioethics and the Humanities. *Addressing Patient-Centered Ethical Issues in Health Care: A Case-Based Study Guide*. Chicago, IL: ASBH, 2017.

American Society for Bioethics and Humanities, "Core Competencies for Healthcare Ethics Consultation." Glenview: IL: American Society for Bioethics and Humanities, 2011.

Andre, Judith. *Bioethics as Practice*. Studies in Social Medicine. Edited by Allan M. Brandt and Larry R. Churchill. Chapel Hill, NC: The University of North Carolina Press, 2002.

Aquinas, Thomas. "Summa Theologiae." 2017. Reprint, Online Edition.

Aristotle. *The Nicomachean Ethics of Aristotle*. https://www.gutenberg.org/files/8438/8438-h/8438-h.htm#chap00.

Arnst, Catherine. "The Best Medical Care in the U.S." *Business Week*, July 17, 2006.

Asch, S. A., E. A. McGlynn, M. M. Hogan, et al. "Comparison of Quality of Care for Patients in the Veterans Health Administration and Patients in a National Sample." *Annals of Internal Medicine* 141, no. 12 (2004): 938–45.

Aultman, Julie, and Cynthia Pathmathasan. "A Call for Diversity and Inclusivity in the Hec-C Program." *The American Journal of Bioethics* 20, no. 3 (2020): 46–50.

Battistella, Edwin L. "What Is the Middle Voice?" In *OUPblog: Oxford University Press's Academic Insights for the Thinking World*. Oxford: Oxford University Press, 2019.

Beauchamp, Tom L. "Reply to Strong on Principlism and Casuistry." *The Journal of Medicine and Philosophy* 25, no. 3 (2000): 342–7.

Bergson, Henri. *Time and Free Will*. Translated by F. L. Pogson. New York: The MacMillan Company, 1913.

Berry, Wendell. "Health Is Membership." Paper presented at the Spirituality and Healing Conference, Louisville, KY, 1994.

Bishop, Jeffrey P. "Ageing and the Technological Imaginary: Living and Dying in the Age of Perpetual Innovation." *Studies in Christian Ethics* 32, no. 1 (2019): 20–35.

Bishop, Jeffrey P. *The Anticipatory Corpse*. Notre Dame, IN: University of Notre Dame Press, 2011.

Bishop, Jeffrey P. "From Anticipatory Corpse to Posthuman God." *Journal of Medicine & Philosophy* 41, no. 6 (2016): 679–95.

Bishop, Jeffrey P. "Intuiting the Excess: Science, Interpretation, and the Transcendence of Life." *Modern Theology* (2025).

Bishop, Jeffrey P. "Of Idolatries and Ersatz Liturgies: The False Gods of Spiritual Assessment." *Christian Bioethics* 19, no. 3 (2013): 332–47.

Bishop, Jeffrey P. "Of Minds and Brains and Cocreation: Psychopharmaceuticals and Modern Technological Imaginaries." *Christian Bioethics: Non-ecumenical Studies in Medical Morality* 24, no. 3 (2018): 224–45.

Bishop, Jeffrey P. "On the Liturgical Consummation of Any Future Enhancement." *Christian Bioethics* 31(2) (2025): 112-120.

Bishop, Jeffrey P. "Principles, Rules, and the Deflation of the Good in Bioethics." *Ethics, Medicine, and Public Health* 3 (2017): 440–51.

Bishop, Jeffrey P. "Technics and Liturgics." *Christian Bioethics: Non-ecumenical Studies in Medical Morality* 26, no. 1 (2020): 12–30.

Bishop, Jeffrey P., Joseph B. Fanning, and Mark J. Bilton. "Echo Calling Narcissus: What Exceeds the Gaze of Clinical Ethics Consultation?" *HEC Forum* 22, no. 1 (2010): 73–84.

Bishop, Jeffrey P., Joseph B. Fanning, and Mark J. Bilton. "Of Goods and Goals and Floundering About: A Dissensus Report on Clinical Ethics Consultation." *HEC Forum* 21, no. 3 (2009): 275–91.

Bliton, Mark J., and Stuart G. Finder. "Strange but Not Stranger: The Peculiar Visage of Philosophy in Clinical Ethics Consultation." *Human Studies* 22 (1999): 69–97.

Boersma, Hans. *Eucharistic Participation: The Reconfiguration of Time and Space*. Vancouver, BC: Regent College Publishing, 2021.

Boersma, Hans. *Heavenly Participation: The Weaving of a Sacramental Tapestry*. Grand Rapids, MI: William B. Eerdmans Publishing Company, 2011.

Bonhoeffer, Dietrich. *Ethics*. Translated by Neville Horton Smith. 1st Touchstone ed. New York: Macmillan Publishing Company, 1955.

Brummett, Abram. "Secular Clinical Ethicists Should Not Be Neutral Toward All Religious Beliefs: An Argument for a Moral-Metaphysical Proceduralism." *The American Journal of Bioethics* 21, no. 6 (2021): 5–16.

Brummett, Abram. "Whose Harm? Which Metaphysic?". *Theoretical Medicine and Bioethics* 40, no. 1 (2019): 43–61.

Brummett, Abram, and Jason T Eberl. "The Many Metaphysical Commitments of Secular Clinical Ethics: Expanding the Argument for a Moral-Metaphysical Proceduralism." *Bioethics* 36, no. 7 (2022): 783–93.

Brummett, Abram, and Christopher J. Ostertag. "Two Troubling Trends in the Conversation over Whether Clinical Ethics Consultants Have Ethics Expertise." *HEC Forum* 30, no. 2 (2018): 157–69.

Brummett, Abram, and E. K. Salter. "Taxonomizing Views of Clinical Ethics Expertise." *American Journal of Bioethics* 19, no. 11 (2019): 50–61.

Buber, Martin. *I and Thou*. Translated by Walter Kaufmann. New York: Charles Scribner's Sons, 1970.

Carr, Brent R. "Side Stepping the Issues: Disappointment with an Ethics Consult for a Medically High Risk Patient." *Narrative Inquiry in Bioethics* 14, no. 1 (2024): 13–16.

Casarett, David J., and Frona Daskal. "The Authority of the Clinical Ethicist." *Hastings Center Report* 28, no. 6 (1998): 6–11.

Chretien, Jean-Louis. *Under the Gaze of the Bible*. Translated by John Marson Dunaway. Perspectives in Continental Philosophy. Edited by John D. Caputo. New York: Fordham University Press, 2015.

Chretien, Jean-Louis. "The Wounded Word: Phenomenology of Prayer." In *Phenomenology and the "Theological Turn": The French Debate*, edited by Dominique Janicaud, Jean-Francois Courtine, Jean-Louis Chretien, Jean-Luc Marion, Michel Henry and Paul Ricoeur, 147–75. New York: Fordham University Press, 2000.

Colgrove, N., and K. K. Evans. "The Place for Religious Content in Clinical Ethics Consultations: A Reply to Janet Malek." *HEC Forum* 31, no. 4 (2019): 305–23.

"Core Competencies for Healthcare Ethics Consultation." Edited by American Society for Bioethics and the Humanities. Glenview, IL: American Society for Bioethics and the Humanities, 2011.

Crenshaw, Kimberle Williams. "Color Blindness, History, and the Law." Chap. 14 In *The House That Race Built*, edited by Wahneema Lubiano, 280–8. New York: Vintage Books, 2010. Reprint, Kindle.

D'souza, Sylvia, and Lucas D. Introna. "Recovering Aristotle's Practice-Based Ontology: Practical Wisdom as Embodied Ethical Intuition." *Journal of Business Ethics* 189, no. 2 (2024): 287–300.

Davison, Andrew. *Participation in God: A Study in Christian Doctrine and Metaphysics.* New York: Cambridge University Press, 2019.
Decrees of the Ecumenical Councils: From Nicaea I to Vatican II. Vol. 1, Washington, DC: Georgetown University Press, 1990.
Dewey, John. *Human Nature and Conduct.* New York: Cosimo Classics, 2007.
Dewey, John. *The Philosophy of John Dewey.* Ed. John J. McDermott. Chicago, IL: University of Chicago Press, 1981.
Dewey, John. *The Political Writings.* Indianapolis, IN: Hackett Publishing Company Inc., 1993.
Dowdy, M. D., C. Robertson, and J. A. Bander. "A Study of Proactive Ethics Consultation for Critically and Terminally Ill Patients with Extended Lengths of Stay." *Critical Care Medicine* 26, no. 11 (1998): 252–9.
Dresser, Rebecca, and John Robertson. "Quality of Life and Non-Treatment Decisions for Incompetent Patients." *Law, Medicine & Healthcare* 17, no. 3 (1989): 234–44.
Dubler, Nancy, and Jeffrey Blustein. "Credentialing Ethics Consultants: An Invitation to Collaboration." *American Journal of Bioethics* 7, no. 2 (2007): 35–7.
Dubler, Nancy, and Carol B. Liebman. *Bioethics Mediation: A Guide to Shaping Shared Solutions.* Rev. and expanded ed. Nashville, TN: Vanderbilt University Press, 2011.
Dubler, Nancy, and Leonard Marcus. *Mediating Bioethical Disputes.* Practical Guide Series. United Hospital Fund, 1994.
Dunne, Joseph. *Back to the Rough Ground: Practical Judgment and the Lure of Technique.* Notre Dame, IN: University of Notre Dame Pess, 1997.
Ellul, Jacques. *The Technological Society.* Translated by John Wilkinson. New York: Vintage Books, 1964.
Emanuel, E. J. and L. L. Emanuel. "Proxy Decision-Making for Incompetent Patients." *JAMA* 267, no. 15 (1992): 2067–71.
Engelhardt, H. Tristram, Jr. *The Foundations of Bioethics.* 2nd ed. Oxford: Oxford University Press, 1996.
Episcopal Church. *The Book of Common Prayer and Administration of the Sacraments and Other Rites and Ceremonies of the Church.* New York: Church Publishing Incorporated, 1789.
Feldman, Sharon L., Sundus H. Riaz, Joshua S. Crites, Jane Jankowski, and Paul J. Ford. "Answering the Call for Standardized Reporting of Clinical Ethics Consultation." *Journal of Clinical Ethics* 31, no. 2 (Summer 2020): 173–7.
Finder, Stuart G., and Mark J. Bliton. *Peer Review, Peer Education, and Modeling in the Practice of Clinical Ethics Consultation: The Zadeh Project.* Cham: Springer Open, 2018.

Fins, J. J., F. G. Miller, and M. D. Bacchetta. "Clinical Pragmatism: Bridging Theory and Practice." *The Kennedy Institute of Ethics Journal* 8, no. 1 (1998): 37–42.

Foucault, Michel. *The Order of Things: An Archaeology of the Human Sciences.* New York: Vintage Books, 1970.

Fox, Ellen, Kenneth Berkowitz, Barbara Chanko, and Tia Powel. *Ethics Consultation: Responding to Ethics Questions in Health Care.* Washington, DC: U.S. Department of Veterans Affairs, 2015, 1–61.

Fox, Ellen, Anita J. Tarzian, Marion Danis, and Christopher Duke. "Ethics Consultation in U.S. Hospitals: Opinions of Ethics Practitioners." *The American Journal of Bioethics* 22, no. 4 (2021): 19–30.

Fox, Ellen, and Jason Adam Wasserman. "Clinical Ethics Fellowship Programs in the United States and Canada: Program Directors' Opinions About Accreditation and Funding." *AJOB Empirical Bioethics* 19, no. 1 (2024): 1–9.

Friedrich, Annie. "The Pitfalls of Proceduralism: An Exploration of the Goods Internal to the Practice of Clinical Ethics Consultation." *HEC Forum* 30, no. 4 (2018): 389–403.

Frolic, Andrea, and Susan B Rubin. "Critical Self-Reflection as Moral Practice: A Collaborative Meditation on Peer Review in Ethics Consultation." In *Peer Review, Peer Education, and Modeling in the Practice of Clinical Ethics Consultation: The Zadeh Project.* Cham: Springer Open, 2018.

Funkenstein, Amos. *Theology and the Scientific Imagination.* Princeton, NJ: Princeton University Press, 1986.

Ganzini, L., L. Volicer, W. Nelson, Ellen Fox, and A. Derse. "Ten Myths About Decision-Making Capacity." *Journal of the American Medical Directors Association* 5 (2004): 263–7.

Gonda, Jan. "Reflections on the Indo-European Medium I." *Lingua* 9 (1961): 30–67.

Grant, George. "Technology and Justice." In *Collected Works of George Grant*, edited by Arthur Davis and Henry Roper, 589–606. Toronto, ON: University of Toronto Press, 2009.

Grimes, Ronald L. *Beginnings in Ritual Studies,* 3rd ed. Waterloo, Canada: Ronald L. Grimes, Ritual Studies International, 2010.

Heidegger, Martin. "Building Dwelling Thinking." Translated by Albert Hofstadter. In *Poetry, Language, Thought.* New York: Harper Colophon Books, 1971.

Heidegger, Martin. "Modern Science, Metaphysics, and Mathematics." Chap. VI In *Basic Writings*, edited by David Farrell Krell. New York: HarperCollins Publishers, 1993.

Heidegger, Martin. "The Question Concerning Technology." In *Basic Writings*. New York, NY: HarperCollins Publishers, 1993.

Heilicser, B. J., D. Meltzer, and Mark Siegler. "The Effect of Clinical Medical Ethics Consultation on Healthcare Costs." *Journal Clinical Ethics* 11, no. 1 (2000): 31–8.

Hemmerle, Klaus. *Theses Towards a Trinitarian Ontology*. Translated by Stephen Churchyard. Brooklyn, NY: Angelico Press, 2020. Thesen zu einer trinitarischen Ontologie in 1976.

Hildegard of Bingen. *Book of Divine Works with Letters and Songs*. Rochester, VT: Bear & Company, 1987.

Ho, Anita. "Relational Autonomy or Undue Pressure? Family's Role in Medical Decision-Making." *Scandanavian Journal of Caring Sciences* 22, no. 1 (2008): 128–35.

Horner, Claire, Andrew Childress, Sophia Fantus, and Janet Malek. "What the Hec-C? An Analysis of the Healthcare Ethics Consultant-Certified Program: One Year In." *American Journal of Bioethics*, no. 3 (2020): 9–18.

Hughes, John. *The End of Work: Theological Critiques of Capitalism*. Illuminations: Theory and Religion. Malden, MA: Blackwell Publishing, 2007.

Hynds, James A., and Joseph A Raho. "A Profession without Expertise? Professionalization in Reverse." *The American Journal of Bioethics* 20, no. 3 (2020): 44–6.

Iltis, Ana Smith. "Bioethics as Methodological Case Resolution: Specification, Specified Principlism and Casuistry." *The Journal of Medicine and Philosophy* 25, no. 3 (2000): 271–84.

Jha, A. K., J. B. Perlin, K. W. Kizer, and R. A. Dudley. "Effects of the Transformation of the Veterans Affairs Health Care System on the Quality of Care." *New England Journal of Medicine* 348, no. 22 (2003): 2218–27.

John of Damascus. *Writings*. Translated by Frederic H. Chase. Washington, DC: Catholic University of America Press, 1958.

Jones, David. *Epoch and Artist*. London: Faber & Faber, 2017.

Jonsen, Albert. "Of Balloons and Bicycles--or--The Relationship between Ethical Theory and Practical Judgment." *Hastings Center Report* 21(5) (1991): 14-16.

Jonsen, Albert R., Mark Siegler, and William J. Winslade. *Clinical Ethics: A Practical Approach to Ethical Decisions in Clinical Medicine*, 9th ed. New York: McGraw Hill, 2022.

Josephson-Storm, Jason Ananda. *Metamodernism: The Future of Theory*. Chicago, IL: University of Chicago Press, 2021.

Kapp, Ernst. *Elements of a Philosophy of Technology: On the Evolutionary History of Culture.* Translated by Lauren Wolfe. Posthumanities. Edited by Cary Wolfe. Minneapolis, MN: University of Minnesota Press, 2018 [1877].

Kornu, Kimbell. "Medical Ersatz Liturgies of Death: Anatomical Dissection and Organ Donation as Biopolitical Practices." *Heythrop Journal* 63, no. 3 (2020): 386–400.

Kotva, Simone. *Effort and Grace: On the Spiritual Exercise of Philosophy.* London: Bloomsbury Publishing, 2020.

Kuczewski, M. "Reconceiving the Family: The Process of Consent in Medical Decision Making." *Hastings Center Report* 26, no. 2 (1996): 30–7.

Kuczewski, Mark G., and Ronald M Polansky. *Bioethics: Ancient Themes in Contemporary Issues.* Cambridge, MA: MIT Press, 2000.

Levinas, Emmanuel. *Is It Righteous to Be? Interviews with Emmanuel Levinas.* Stanford, CA: Stanford University Press, 2001.

Lewin, David. "The Middle Voice in Eckhart and Modern Continental Philosophy." *Medieval Mystical Theology* 20, no. 1 (2011): 28–46.

Lewis, C S. *The Weight of Glory.* New York: Harper Collins, 2001.

MacIntyre, Alasdair. *After Virtue: A Study in Moral Theory.* Notre Dame: University of Notre Dame Press, 1981.

MacIntyre, Alasdair *Three Rival Versions of Moral Enquiry: Encyclopaedia, Genealogy, and Tradition: Being Gifford Lectures Delivered in the University of Edinburgh in 1988.* Notre Dame, IN: University of Notre Dame Press, 1990.

MacIntyre, Alasdair. *Whose Justice? Which Rationality?* Notre Dame, IN: University of Notre Dame Press, 1988.

Macklin, Ruth. *Against Relativism: Cultural Diversity and the Search for Ethical Universals in Medicine.* Oxford: Oxford University Press, 1999.

Mason, Jordan. "Confessional Approach to Disclosure of Medical Error." *Christian Bioethics* 27, no. 2 (2021): 203–22.

Mason, Jordan. "Techniques of Ordering and the Dynamism of Being: A Critique of Standardized Clinical Ethics Consultation Methods." *HEC Forum* 35 (2022): 253–69.

Mason, Jordan. "Transhumanism, Motion, and Human Perfection." *Christian Bioethics* 28, no. 3 (2022): 185–96.

McGee, Glenn. "Phronesis in Clinical Ethics." *Theoretical Medicine* 17 (1996): 317–28.

Meilaender, Gilbert. *Body, Soul, and Bioethics.* Notre Dame, IN: University of Notre Dame Press, 1995.

Milbank, John. *Theology and Social Theory: Beyond Secular Reason*, 2nd ed. Malden, MA: Blackwell Publishing, 2006.

Milbank, John, Catherine Pickstock, and Graham Ward, eds. *Radical Orthodoxy: A New Theology*. London: Routledge, 1999.

Miller, Franklin G., Joseph J. Fins, and Matthew D. Bacchetta. "Clinical Pragmatism: John Dewey and Clinical Ethics." *Journal of Contemporary Health Law & Policy* 13, no. 1 (1996): 27–51.

Moreno, Jonathan. *Deciding Together: Bioethics and Moral Consensus*. Oxford: Oxford University Press, 1995.

Morreim, Haavi. "Mediating in Healthcare's Clinical Setting: Time for a Course Correction." *Ohio State Journal on Dispute Resolution* 35, no. 1 (2019): 81–108.

Moyse, Ashley. *Reading Karl Barth, Interrupting Moral Technique, Transforming Biomedical Ethics*. Content and Context in Theological Ethics. Edited by Mary Jo Iozzio. London: Palgrave Macmillan, 2015.

Moyse, Ashley John. *The Art of Living for a Technological Age*. Dispatches: Turning Points in Theology and Global Crises. Edited by Ashley John Moyse and Scott A. Kirkland. Minneapolis, MN: Fortress Press, 2021.

Moyse, Ashley John. "Malek's Programmatic Secularism? A Dissent." *Christian Bioethics* 28, no. 2 (2022): 99–108.

Oliver, Simon. *Creation: A Guide for the Perplexed*. Guides for the Perplexed. London: Bloomsbury, 2017.

Ong, Walter J. *Orality and Literacy: The Technologizing of the Word*. New York: Routledge, 2002 [1982].

Opel, Douglas J., Dena Brownstein, Douglas S. Diekema, Benjamin S. Wilfond, and Robert A. Pearlman. "Integrating Ethics and Patient Safety: The Role of Clinical Ethics Consultants in Quality Improvement." *The Journal of Clinical Ethics* 20, no. 3 (2009): 220–7.

Orr, Robert, and Wayne Shelton. "A Process and Format for Clinical Ethics Consultation." *The Journal of Clinical Ethics* 20, no. 1 (Spring 2009): 1–11.

Pellegrino, Edmund D. "Bioethics at Century's Turn: Can Normative Ethics Be Retrieved?" *Journal of Medicine & Philosophy* 25, no. 6 (2000): 655–75.

Pellegrino, Edmund D. *The Philosophy of Medicine Reborn: A Pellegrino Reader*. Notre Dame, IN: University of Notre Dame Pess, 2008.

Pellegrino, Edmund D. "Professing Medicine, Virtue Based Ethics, and the Retrieval of Professionalism." In *Working Virtue: Virtue Ethics and Contemporary Moral Problems*, edited by Rebecca L Walker and Philip J Ivanhoe, 61–86. Oxford: Oxford Academic, 2007.

Pellegrino, Edmund D., and David C. Thomasma. *The Christian Virtues in Medical Practice*. Washington, DC: Georgetown University Press, 1996.

Pellegrino, Edmund D., and David C. Thomasma. *The Virtues in Medical Practice*. New York: Oxford University Press, 1993.

Pickstock, Catherine. *After Writing: On the Liturgical Consummation of Philosophy*. Challenges in Contemporary Theology. Edited by Gareth Jones and Lewis Ayres. Oxford: Blackwell Publishers, 1998.

Pickstock, Catherine. *Aspects of Truth: A New Religious Metaphysics*. Cambridge: Cambridge University Press, 2020.

Pickstock, Catherine. *Repetition and Identity*. The Literary Agenda. Oxford: Oxford University Press, 2013.

Post, Linda, Jeffrey Blustein, and Nancy Dubler. "The Doctor-Proxy Relationship: An Untapped Resource." *Journal of Law, Medicine & Ethics* 27, no. 1 (1999): 5–12.

Rasmussen, Lisa M. "Non-Certain Foundations: Clinical Ethics Consultation for the Rest of Us." In *At the Foundations of Bioethics and Biopolitics: Critical Essays on the Thought of H. Tristram Engelhardt, Jr.*, edited by Lisa M. Rasmussen, Ana Iltis and Mark J. Cherry, 187–99. Cham: Springer International Publishing, 2015.

Rasmussen, Lisa M., A. S. Iltis, and M. J. Cherry. *At the Foundations of Bioethics and Biopolitics: Critical Essays on the Thought of H. Tristram Engelhardt, Jr.* Springer International Publishing, 2015. doi:10.1007/978-3-319-18965-9.

Rodeheffer, Jane Kelley. "Practical Reasoning in Medicine and the Rise of Clinical Ethics." *The Journal of Clinical Ethics* 1, no. 3 (1990): 187–92.

Saint Bonaventure. *Holiness of Life*. London: Forgotten Books, 2018. Classic.

Saint Bonaventure. *The Works of Bonaventure: Cardinal Seraphic Doctor and Saint: Volume I. Mystical Opuscula*. Translated by Jose de Vinck. Quick Time Press, 2020.

Saint Maximus the Confessor. *On the Ecclesiastical Mystagogy*. Translated by Jonathan J. Armstrong. Popular Patristics Series. Edited by John Behr. Yonkers, NY: St. Vladimir's Seminary Press, 2019.

Schneiderman, L. J., T. Gilmer, and H. D. Teetzel. "Impact of Ethics Consultations in the Intensive Care Setting: A Randomized, Controlled Trial." *Critical Care Medicine* 28, no. 12 (2000): 3920–4.

Schneiderman, L. J., T. Gilmer, H. D. Teetzel, et al. "Effect of Ethics Consultations on Nonbeneficial Life-Sustaining Treatments in the Intensive Care Setting: A Randomized Controlled Trial." *JAMA* 290, no. 9 (2003): 1166–72.

Schumann, John H., and David Alfandre. "Clinical Ethical Decision Making: The Four Topics Approach." *Seminars in Medical Practice* 11 (2008): 36–42.

Scofield, G. R. "Ethics Consultation: The Least Dangerous Profession?" *Cambridge Quarterly of Healthcare Ethics* 2, no. 4 (Fall 1993): 417–26.

Secundy, Marian Gray. "Thinking About Clinical Ethics." *American Journal of Bioethics* 1, no. 4 (2001): 59.

Shapin, Steven, and Simon Schaffer. *Leviathan and the Air-Pump: Hobbes, Boyle, and the Experimental Life.* Princeton, NJ: Princeton University Press, 1985.

Shelton, Wayne N., and Bruce D. White. "The Process to Accredit Clinical Ethics Fellowship Programs Should Start Now." *The American Journal of Bioethics* 16, no. 3 (2016): 28–30.

Siegert, Bernhard. *Cultural Techniques: Grids, Filters, Doors, and Other Articulations of the Real.* Translated by Geoffrey Winthrop-Young. New York: Fordham University Press, 2015.

Sigurdson, Ola. *Heavenly Bodies: Incarnation, the Gaze, and Embodiment in Christian Theology.* Translated by Carl Olsen. Grand Rapids, MI: William B. Eerdmans Publishing Company, 2016.

Simmons, J. Aaron, and Bruce Benson. *The New Phenomenology.* New York: Bloomsbury Academic, 2013.

Smith, James K. A. *Awaiting the Kingdom: Reforming Public Theology.* Cultural Liturgies. Edited by James K. A. Smith. Grand Rapids, MI: Baker Academic, 2017.

Smith, James K. A. *Desiring the Kingdom: Worship, Worldview, and Cultural Formation.* Cultural Liturgies. Edited by James K. A. Smith. Grand Rapids, MI: Baker Academic, 2009.

Smith, James K. A. *Imagining the Kingdom: How Worship Works.* Cultural Liturgies. Edited by James K. A. Smith. Grand Rapids, MI: Baker Academic, 2013.

Smith, James K. A. *You Are What You Love: The Spiritual Power of Habit.* Grand Rapids, MI: Brazos Press, 2016.

Smith, Mark M. *Sensing the Past: Seeing, Hearing, Smelling, Tasting, and Touching in History.* Berkeley, CA: University of California Press, 2008.

Stiegler, Bernard. *Technics and Time, 1: The Fault of Epimetheus.* Translated by Richard Beardsworth and George Collins. Redwood City, CA: Stanford University Press, 1998.

Stiegler, Bernard. *Technics and Time, 2: Disorientation.* Translated by Stephen Barker. Redwood City, CA: Stanford University Press, 2008.

Stiegler, Bernard. *Technics and Time, 3: Cinematic Time and the Question of Malaise.* Translated by Stephen Barker. Redwood City, CA: Stanford University Press, 2010.

Svenaeus, Fredrik. "Hermeneutics of Medicine in the Wake of Gadamer." *Theoretical Medicine and Bioethics* 24:5 (2003), 407–431.

Taylor, Charles. *A Secular Age*. Cambridge: Belknap Press, 2007.
Taylor, Neil. "Derrida's 'Middle Voice': Writing as *Difference* and the Textual 'Limits' of Our World." University of Sussex, 1997.
The Clinical Ethics Consultation Benchmarking Collaborative. https://cecbc.net.
Thomasma, David C. "Virtue Theory in Philosophy of Medicine." In *Handbook of Bioethics: Taking Stock of the Field from a Philosophical Perspective*, edited by George Khushf, 89–120. Dordrecht: Springer Netherlands, 2004.
Thompson, Dennis F. "What Is Practical Ethics?" In *Ethics at Harvard 1907-2007*, edited by The President and Fellows of Harvard College, 5–7. Harvard University Edmond J. Safra Foundation Center for Ethics, 2007.
Thomson, Iain. *Heidegger on Ontotheology*. Cambridge: Cambridge University Press, 2005.
Thoreau, Henry David. *Walden*. Boston, MA: Ticknor and Fields, 1854. https://archive.org/details/waldenorlifei00thor/page/40/mode/2up?q=%22their+tools%22.
Toulmin, Stephen. "The Tyranny of Principles." *Hastings Center Report* 11(6) (1982): 31–9.
Tristram Engelhardt, H. "Credentialing Strategically Ambiguous and Heterogeneous Social Skills: The Emperor without Clothes." *HEC Forum*, no. 3 (2009): 293–306.
Verbeek, Peter-Paul. *Moralizing Technology: Understanding and Designing the Morality of Things*. Chicago, IL: University of Chicago Press, 2011.
Verbeek, Peter-Paul. "Obstetric Ultrasound and the Technological Mediation of Morality: A Postphenomenological Analysis." *Human Studies* 31, no. 1 (2008): 11–26.
Walker, Margaret Urban. "Keeping Moral Space Open." *Hastings Center Report* 23, no. 2 (1993): 33–40.
Williams, Rowan. *Christ the Heart of Creation*. London: Bloomsbury Continuum, 2018.
Wolfe, Judith. *Heidegger and Theology*. Philosophy and Theology Series. London: Bloomsbury T&T Clark, 2014.
Yannaras, Christos. *Relational Ontology*. Translated by Norman Russell. Brookline, MA: Holy Cross Orthodox Press, 2011.
Yoon, Nicholas Yue Shuen, Yun Ting Ong, Hong Wei Yap, Kuang Teck Tay, Elijah Gin Lim, Clarissa Wei Shuen Cheong, Wei Qiang Lim, et al. "Evaluating Assessment Tools of the Quality of Clinical Ethics Consultations: A Systematic Scoping Review from 1992 to 2019." *BMC Medical Ethics* 21, no. 1 (2020): 51.

Zaborowski, Holger. "Technology, Truth, and Thinking: Martin Heidegger's Reading of Ernst Junger's the Worker." Chap. 8 In *Hiedegger's Question of Being: Dasein, Truth, and History*, 165–83. Washington, DC: The Catholic University of America Press, 2017.

Zaner, Richard M. *The Context of Self: A Phenomenological Inquiry Using Medicine as a Clue.* Athens, OH: Ohio University Press, 1981.

Zaner, Richard M. *Ethics and the Clinical Encounter.* Englewood Cliffs, NJ: Prentice Hall, 1988.

Zaner, Richard M. "Is 'Ethicist' Anything to Call a Philosopher?" *Human Studies* 7 (1984): 71–90.

Zaner, Richard M., ed. *Performance, Talk, Reflection: What Is Going on in Clinical Ethics Consultation?* Dordrecht: Kluwer, 1999.

Zizioulas, John D. *Being as Communion.* Contemporary Greek Theologians. Edited by Kallistos of Diokleia Christos Yannaras, Costa Carras. Crestwood, NY: St. Vladimir's Seminary Press, 1985.

Index

American Society for Bioethics and Humanities (ASBH)   17, 62–5, 73–5, 171–9
analogia entis   31–3, 103, 138–9, 148–50

Bioethics Mediation (Dubler and Liebman)   25 n.60, 62–74, 100
Bishop, Jeffrey P
   clinical ethics   8, 119, 131 n.32
   and Foucault   102, 106
Boersma, Hans   138–41
Bonhoeffer, Dietrich   36–7, 167
bringing-forth, *see poiesis*
Buber, Martin   15

CASES Method   75–84
challenging-forth
   in Bioethics Mediation   73
   in CASES Method   76–7, 83–4
   in Clinical Pragmatism   55–9
   definition   6–7
   in Four Boxes Method   49, 51–4
   and standardization   13–20, 33–6, 39–42
Clinical Pragmatism (Miller, Fins, and Bacchetta)   55–62
cultural liturgies   41

Dewey, John   55–58, 61–2

Ellul, Jacques   10–12, 47–9, 51–3, 74
encounter   36–9
   and liturgy   136–7
   and phenomenology (Zaner)   93–8, 101–2, 107
   and practical ethics   28, 117, 120, 123, 163–4
enframing   17–18, 98
ersatz liturgies
   definition   42, 39–42

   methods as   48, 54, 60, 67, 83, 108, 167–8
Ethics Facilitation   25 n.60, 73–5
eucharistic liturgy   40, 139–50, 160, 171
evaluation of techniques   124–8

Foucault, Michel, *see* Kant, Immanuel
Four Boxes Method (Jonsen, Siegler, and Winslade)   48–54

gaze
   vs. behold   37, 117–19, 164–5, 179
   and philosophy of technology   5–9, 15–16
   and standardized techniques   16–17, 54

Heidegger, Martin   3–18, 35–6
Hemmerle, Klaus   138, 143, 146–9

I-Thou relationship   15, 144

Kant, Immanuel   38–9
   Foucault's critique of   102–6
Kapp, Ernst (1808–1896)   8–9
Kornu, Kimbell, *see ersatz* liturgies

liturgical stance   126, 137, 152, 159–69, 171–9

Maximus the Confessor   147, 149
middle voice   117–19
   in clinical ethics consultation   151–2, 160, 164–6, 178–9
mode of revealing   4–6
Moyse, Ashley John   14–15, 69, 166, *see also* techno-ontology

New phenomenology   36–9
non-identical repetition   28–36

Ong, Walter (1912–2003) 9

participatory ontology 31–4, 138–53, 169
Phenomenological Method (Zaner) 93–102, 105–9, 115, 120, 163
phenomenology 36–9, 93–109
phronesis 120, 121–4
Pickstock, Catherine 12, 28–31, 140–51
poiesis 6, 13, 16–17, 20, 42, 116, 124, 137
practical ethics
    definition 115–21
    vs. pragmatism 55–7
    three questions of 120, 123, 152
professionalization of clinical ethics 64–5, 73–5

Scotus, Duns 30, 31–2, 103, 143
Smith, James K. A. 41
standardization
    of clinical ethics as a profession 64–5, 78–9
    of individual methods 47–84, *see also* challenging forth
    of technique in clinical ethics 13–20, 27–8, 40–1, *see also* challenging forth

techne 3–16, 31, 119, 123, 125, 138
techno-ontology 13–15, 33–6, 166–7

univocity of being 29–36

Verbeek, Peter-Paul 9–10
virtue ethics of medicine (Pellegrino and Thomasma) 121–4

William of Ockham 31–2, 103
Williams, Rowan 145–7

Zizioulas, John 140–50

About the Author

Jordan Mason is a theologian and healthcare ethicist based in Santa Rosa, California. She holds a master of divinity from McAfee School of Theology at Mercer University and a PhD in theology and healthcare ethics from Saint Louis University. Her areas of interest include theological bioethics, liturgical theology, and the philosophy of technology. She has published on wide-ranging topics such as the professionalization of clinical ethics, organ transplantation, medical error, and dementia. Jordan is currently a practicing clinical ethicist for Providence St. Joseph Health in Northern California, where she serves six hospitals.